MAKING SENSE OF YOUR MEDICAL CAREER

MAKING SENSE OF YOUR MEDICAL CAREER

YOUR STRATEGIC GUIDE TO SUCCESS

Riaz Agha BSc(Hons)
Final-year medical student, Guy's, King's and
St Thomas' School of Medicine, London, UK;
Founder and Managing Editor,
International Journal of Surgery

Editorial Advisors

Sir Graeme Catto MD, FRCP, FRSE
Pro Vice-Chancellor for Medicine, University of London;
Vice-Principal, King's College London, UK

Sir Barry Jackson MS, FRCS, FRCP
Past President of the Royal Society of Medicine in London;
Past President of the Royal College of Surgeons of England, UK

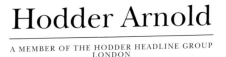

Hodder Arnold

A MEMBER OF THE HODDER HEADLINE GROUP
LONDON

First published in Great Britain in 2005 by
Hodder Education, a member of the Hodder Headline Group,
338 Euston Road, London NW1 3BH

http://www.hoddereducation.co.uk

Distributed in the United States of America by
Oxford University Press Inc.,
198 Madison Avenue, New York, NY10016
Oxford is a registered trademark of Oxford University Press

Whilst the advice and information in this book are believed to be true and
accurate at the date of going to press, neither the author[s] nor the publisher
can accept any legal responsibility or liability for any errors or omissions
that may be made. In particular (but without limiting the generality of the
preceding disclaimer), every effort has been made to check drug dosages;
however, it is still possible that errors have been missed. Furthermore,
dosage schedules are constantly being revised and new side-effects
recognized. For these reasons the reader is strongly urged to consult the
drug companies' printed instructions before administering any of the drugs
recommended in this book.

British Library Cataloguing-in-Publication Data
A catalogue record for this book is available from the British Library

Library of Congress Cataloging-in-Publication Data
A catalog record for this book is available from the Library of Congress

ISBN-10: 0 340 88737 0
ISBN-13: 978 0 340 88737 0

1 2 3 4 5 6 7 8 9 10

Commissioning editor: Joanna Koster
Project editor: Heather Smith
Production controller: Jane Lawrence
Cover design: Georgina Hewitt

Typeset in 10.5/13 Rotis Serif by Charon Tec Pvt. Ltd, Chennai, India
Printed and bound in Italy

What do you think about this book? Or any other Hodder Arnold
title? Please visit our website at www.hoddereducation.co.uk

This book is dedicated to all the hard-working lecturers, doctors and students who have helped to inspire me over the years. A special thanks goes to my family who have supported me throughout my entire life.

ABOUT THE AUTHOR

After being awarded 4 A's at A-level in 1998, Riaz went to work for Harrods in Knightsbridge, London, for 1 year before entering Guy's, King's and St Thomas' School of Medicine (GKT). There he was awarded the Pre-Clinical Scholarship, the Distinction in Basic Medical Sciences, a 1st in his intercalated BSc(Hons) in Anatomy and 20 academic prizes and awards.

Throughout medical school, Riaz has been engaged in a variety of research projects both at GKT and at Harvard University, with many going on to be formally published in peer-reviewed journals and presented at international scientific meetings. He has also worked as a Student Ambassador for King's College London, as a Medical Secretary and as the PA to the Manager of the Surgical Directorate in a major London Hospital.

As an advisor to the Student BMJ and as a member of the local BMA Committee, Riaz has been engaged in a breadth of student issues. After becoming President of the Guy's, King's and St Thomas' Surgical Society, which under his leadership became the largest student surgical society in the UK, he was awarded the Gold Medal by the King's College London Student's Union. Riaz has also served on the board of the Section of Plastic Surgery at the Royal Society of Medicine in London and as an invited reviewer for the 39th edition of *Gray's Anatomy*.

In 2003, Riaz founded Surgical Associates Ltd and became its sole Director. Later in that year he launched the International Journal of Surgery, which is now published by Elsevier with Riaz remaining the Owner and Managing Editor.

CONTENTS

CONTRIBUTORS

Mohammad Al-Ubaydli MB BChir MA Cantab
Bethesda, MD, USA;
Author of *Handheld Computers for Doctors*
(John Wiley and Sons Ltd, 2003)

Georgina Bentliff MA BSc(Hons)
Publisher, London, UK

Martin Hewitt BA PG Dip Inf
Information Specialist, King's College London, London, UK

Carole Hjelm BSc PhD
King's College London Careers Service, London, UK

Sonia Hutton-Taylor MBBS FRCS FRCOphth DO
Founder, Medical Forum, Overton, UK

FOREWORD

We have no doubt that any medical student would benefit
from reading this book, and so would many of their teachers.
It was conceived and edited by a medical student for the
benefit of other medical students. All the chapters address
topics of real and continuing interest for today's
undergraduates, and some sections will be of use to
postgraduates as well. Views are expressed clearly and
succinctly; concepts are explored lucidly and, when offered,
the advice is relevant to current circumstances, with
appropriate recommendations for further reading and details
of useful websites.

The text emphasizes the competitive aspects of a career in
medicine, providing ideas and strategies on how students can
maximize their time at medical school and thus make more
effective applications afterwards. The potential advantages and
disadvantages of any particular decision are often considered
from the perspective of enhancing the student's distinctiveness
and to give them a competitive edge. Although some of us
continue to believe that students are motivated by the thrill of
learning, we believe that this book provides just the right
balance of insight and pragmatism that will appeal to many
students. It is a remarkable achievement and we believe that it

justly merits a place on the student's personal bookshelf as well as in libraries everywhere.

Sir Graeme Catto MD, FRCP, FRSE
Pro Vice-Chancellor for Medicine, University of London
Vice-Principal, King's College London

Sir Barry Jackson MS, FRCS, FRCP
Past President of the Royal Society of Medicine in London
Past President of the Royal College of Surgeons of England

PREFACE

For a medical student life can be easy: turn up at lectures and clinics and simply go with the flow. Five or six years later it hits you: can you really get a job in that specialty? A career in medicine, like any other high-flying professional career, is highly competitive, which inherently means some people fail to realize their ambitions. The Royal College of Surgeons of England states that for some posts up to 200 people apply. Certain specialties are more competitive than others, but in general competition is set to increase and is worst in London. According to the Department of Health, the number of medical students in England increased by 57% between 1997 and 2001, and then by 28% from 2000 to 2003; according to the BMA there are now 22,500 medical students across 30 medical schools (October 2004) in the UK. This increase has not been matched by a proportionate increase in training posts, with many specialties having 5–10 eligible candidates per post nationally.

This level of competition is fierce, and medical students often do not receive the structured careers advice, mentoring or support they need to deal with it. Students therefore seek advice from individual consultants or more senior students. Such advice is inherently biased and does not provide a balanced portfolio of information from which to make informed decisions. Rather, a rushed opinion is provided which is vague, lacking in detail, and which can be to the detriment of the student's future. Your career and your life are worth more than fleeting comments in corridors or 'snap' e-mails.

This book aims to help you make the most of your time at medical school, providing you with the high-quality information you need to build a successful career in the specialty that you want to pursue. It will tell you what potential employers are looking for on your CV, how you can go about fulfilling their criteria and ultimately how to get shortlisted and then selected for competitive posts. Additionally, the book will guide you through the most important decisions you will make while at medical school, such as whether do to an intercalated BSc, where to go on elective and how to get funding for both of these. You will also learn how to obtain the relevant skills you need to become a well-rounded professional, so that you can be a more effective twenty-first-century clinician. The book is also fully supported by an accompanying website at www.yourmedicalcareer.com.

Riaz Agha
2005

ACKNOWLEDGEMENTS

The author would like to extend special thanks to the following people for being an incredible source of inspiration and guidance:

Dr Paul Brown
Sir Graeme Catto
Sir Barry Jackson
Dr Alistair Hunter
Mrs Barbara Webb
Dr Chris Reid
Dr Dennis Orgill
Professor David Cooper
Dr Mohammad Al-Ubaydli
Professor Susan Standring
Professor Harold Ellis
Dr Derek Cooper
Dr David Green
Professor Michael Baum
Professor Gwyn Williams
Professor the Lord McColl
Mr David Ross
Professor Irving Benjamin
Sir Peter Morris
Professor Edward Howard
Mr Gordon Muir
Mr Munir Ahmed

1

CAREER BUILDING STARTS IN THE MIND

Riaz Agha

In order to beat the competition and become successful, you need to make yourself (and your CV) stand out. This process must start in your mind, as you need to change the way you think. Often in medicine, we are told what to do and spoon-fed facts about diseases, which we memorize for the purposes of passing exams (a large proportion being forgotten straight afterwards). This seemingly never-ending cycle can place your mind into a groove that lacks creative thought – it has become geared towards taking on new information, rather than constructing new ideas and being innovative. This is not ideal for manoeuvring yourself into a position from which you can launch successful applications for competitive jobs and achieve your ultimate goals in life. Let us consider some of the key concepts involved in changing the way you think.

ENTREPRENEURSHIP

As a priority, you must reactivate the creative part of your mind and become an entrepreneur. You need to start looking for career-building opportunities both within and outside your medical school. Such opportunities may include positions on committees, setting up a journal club or a society, writing a book, doing research projects which will lead to publications, international presentations, and so on. The opportunities to differentiate yourself are limited only by your imagination. An entrepreneur is often defined by their ability to leverage resources beyond their control: in your case, this may involve discussions with family, friends and tutors to see what opportunities they can present you with.

Such a discussion with my personal tutor led to me joining his research team over the summer, for which I secured funding from the Wellcome Trust. As a result, I became one of the authors on a scientific paper and gained important laboratory skills and experience. This experience was subsequently vital in obtaining a place at Harvard to do research for my elective (for which I received 13 awards and gained scientific publications and presentations on international platforms). One achievement led to another. However, such a cascade would have been almost impossible to predict at the start. This brings me to the next key concept: you need to learn to develop yourself generically, as you never know where things may lead.

DEVELOP YOURSELF

In order to develop yourself, you need to think of yourself as a company or even a share on the stock market, e.g. Riaz Agha Ltd. Good companies anywhere in the world value their staff and spend large sums on training them in specific knowledge, skills and attitudes. In fact, many hire professional headhunters to actively seek out people with the attributes they are looking for – millions are spent each year on the acquisition of the right people with the right 'mix' of abilities.

I deliberately went about trying to get laboratory experience early on at medical school, as I knew it would help to keep my options open and raise my value in the 'marketplace' (ultimately it was used as leverage to secure the elective that I really wanted to do). Further down the line, I realized just how important it was to know statistics for the purposes of research (and discussing research methods competently with others). I decided to get one-to-one tuition with a statistician working at my university: again, this proved critical to a string of research projects which followed, as well as my ability to critically analyse scientific papers at the Harvard Research Meetings while on elective.

In this way, you need to take charge of yourself and actively manage your personal development, select the skills you want to acquire, especially those that you know will be useful in your future career, and go about getting the relevant experience. In any case, it is a very good idea to expand your skill set, whether it be teaching, managerial, research, statistics, etc., and learn new techniques and thought processes at every opportunity.

NETWORKING

In order to access as many opportunities as possible, you need to network. In other words, you need to build relationships with a wider set of key people. Such people may be in a position to offer you placements, opportunities and advice. They may also be able to support some of your projects and provide you with key contacts. In order to get others to work for *you* on developing *your* projects/ideas, you will need to demonstrate your leadership skills, in other words creating and communicating a plausible vision and empowering and motivating colleagues so they can help you achieve it.

Networking also applies to organizations: go to the websites for the Royal Society of Medicine, the Royal Colleges and other professional associations; attend meetings that interest you and talk to people who attend – tell them you are a medical student looking for advice on how to improve your chances of getting into their specialty. The answers can be very different and may not be helpful, but you are building up your set of contacts all the time, and this is vital.

Networking also helps to raise your profile, which means you will be on the radar screen when the right opportunities come along. It will also enable you to build a parallel career in another industry altogether. For example, your main career may be as a plastic surgeon, but you may also have a parallel career in:

- Publishing – writing books, developing websites, working for journal editorial boards and writing pieces for broadsheets and other health media.
- Medical broadcasting and radio.
- Business – developing wound care devices which you bring to the market via your own surgical devices company.
- Consultancy – to major companies that want your advice on how they can improve their implants or other medical devices.
- Non-executive director positions on company boards – later in your career.
- Medicopolitical – as an adviser to medical defence companies on aspects of litigation.

Self-marketing requires a three-pronged strategy: speak, write and network. Joining the right professional groups/committees and gaining external recognition is important. You must, however, be good at what you do: marketing terrible work often leads to a short career. Participate in those extra activities that you find personally and professionally fulfilling, and never try to give the impression you are pursuing something just for the purposes of exposure. Networking, keeping a broad mind, developing generic skills and learning about a parallel career that interests you is a good start towards a varied and fulfilling career.

DEVELOP A STRATEGY

Once you have started to think differently, you need to move towards harnessing your creative energies for the purposes of real action. This requires a number of processes:

- Development of a strategy – deciding what you want to do.
- Defining your objectives – what do you want to achieve? You should be able to see your goals clearly, and these should be specific, written down, and have a date on them.

- Understand where you are now – what have you achieved already; if appropriate, compare your performance with those around you and find out how they achieve certain things better.
- What are your priorities?
- Develop your implementation plan – lay out the steps involved in achieving your objectives.

The execution of your implementation plan will also help you: develop a sense of timing (to capture opportunities); to be able to make decisions quickly based on intuition; to understand risk and reward; to be a sales person and to bring key people on to your projects (and keep them onboard); to develop your people skills; to create a variety of project streams (you can choose which you wish to work on at any particular time, and all can pay dividends for your career). You will also learn to be comfortable with uncertainty.

MOTIVATION AND DRIVE

Ultimately, in order to stay focused and continue building yourself and your career, you need motivation and drive. The way to maintain these is to remind yourself of the reasons for working so hard in the first place, what your goals are and how difficult it is to achieve them. Always manage your time efficiently and work smarter, not just harder (see Chapter 2, Time Management).

As you start to achieve greater success in your time at medical school, you will start to enjoy the thrill of chasing your objectives. Developing yourself and your career adds variety to your life, and it can be immensely fulfilling to unlock your potential as well as realizing your career ambitions.

PART

I

GETTING THE SKILLS YOU NEED

2

HOW TO MANAGE YOUR TIME, FINANCES AND STRESS

Riaz Agha

The skills of good time, financial and stress management are crucial to success in life. Whenever you have a problem in any of these three areas the solution is broadly the same: assess the situation, set and implement an agenda for change, and regain control. Of course, primary prevention will always be better than cure.

TIME MANAGEMENT

Priorities and motivation

Successful time management starts in the mind – it has to come from within and result in consistent self-discipline. You need to establish what your overall goals are and then set your agenda to allow you achieve them (or to achieve steps in their direction). You need to differentiate between urgent, important and routine tasks: prioritizing can become difficult when there are too many items on your list, and as a result you end up losing focus. Work through your 'to do' list and refer back to the underlying motivation for each of your goals to remind yourself just how important they are – this will help you prioritize.

Relationships

Other people are often the key manipulators of your time: they swing the balance between your getting ahead, staying on schedule or getting behind. You need to identify the instances of the latter, such as conversations in corridors and on the phone which are of little significance, and try and minimize them. You need to strike a balance between friendly conversation to maintain key relationships and the need to get on with important tasks to help you achieve your goals (and to prevent you getting stressed later over how little you have achieved so far that day).

Remember the delicate balance of such personal relationships: what is the person asking from you; what do they have to gain; are their gains greater than your benefits/costs; would they be willing to help you in the future; do they have key skills you need, and so on (who is playing chess better)? These calculations often happen subconsciously, but you can be more efficient if you bring them to the front of your mind.

Procrastination

Also known as 'the thief of time', this also comes from within and must be dealt with from within. Procrastination can be thought of as an internally driven avoidance behaviour: it may be rooted in fear of failure, rebellion, an expression of resentment due to lack of control, and so on. Break the cycle by setting clear priorities (you should always be able to visualize your goals very clearly) and doing difficult tasks when you are at your most fresh (be that morning or evening). If you have a 'mental block', divide complex tasks into smaller, more manageable ones. Don't let them build up on you, and remember that things will only get worse if you put them off.

The magnitude of the task can be frightening, especially if it has built up over time. Before starting, it is important to have a think about the best aspects of completing the task, rather than the more adverse ones (i.e. what will it do for your career, rather than it being boring and time consuming). Avoid rationalizing your procrastination – e.g. 'all work and no play. . . .'; if you realize you are doing this, also realize that your life is not just about a phrase and that you are not governed by myths or arbitrary rules. Your competitors will no doubt be getting on with their task list: do you really want to give in so easily and let them win?

As well as breaking the task into smaller components, you should 'start low and slow' (i.e. start with the easiest components of the task to give yourself a run-up to the more difficult parts). The next step is to prepare to get started: clean your desk, your room, and perhaps talk to others for information on the task. This will lead into first step, which is often the hardest: you may even start the task without even realizing it! Furthermore, once you start, you realize it wasn't actually as bad as you thought.

One key thing to bear in mind when dealing with procrastination is that you only live once: do you really want to score an 'own goal' with your life? If not, take back control and apply yourself. If the worst comes to the worst and you just feel too low to do anything, do something more active, such as taking some exercise: it will clear your mind, release some feel-good endorphins, and will benefit your health in any case, so you are still making progress and you didn't waste any time in 'analysis paralysis'. You are now ready to take on that task and the momentum is with you. Remember, you have the ultimate choice about your own goals and whether you choose to achieve them (and how). Finally, once you have completed the task, remember to reward yourself with those pleasurable activities that were previously your excuse for not working. Now, think to yourself just how much more fulfilling these activities can be when you don't have work hanging over your 'good time'.

Reading

This can take up vast amounts of time and so you need to be efficient. Ask yourself why you are reading this and what are you trying to gain – what are the key questions you want answered? or are you simply 'skimming' for something interesting? You can waste time reading pages of text to find out that you only needed to read two or three lines near the end or somewhere in the middle to get the key pieces of information you were looking for. Skim through sections and look for key words – quite literally, speed-read across the entire page. You don't have to read every word or go through every chapter – make the book work for you, not the other way around.

For a book, read the blurb, the chapter list and the introduction, and then go to the chapter you are interested in. For journal papers, read the abstract and the introduction, skim the methods and results (look at the tables and graphs), and then read the discussion. However, there may be times when you need to pay careful attention to methodology and the presentation of the results, especially when you are doing research or critical analysis for a journal club, so always remember what your objectives are in the first place.

Practical steps for effective time management

- Set clear goals and priorities, as vague ones increase procrastination.
- Don't insist everything is high priority: make sure you are in the right mood to make such decisions. If you feel low, do something morale boosting and then build your task list and prioritize.
- At the start of each day make a list of 'things to do' or objectives for that day. If you don't complete a particular task, carry it over to the next day until it is complete. At the end of each day, plan for tomorrow.
- Don't lose sight of your objectives – store them ideally on a pocket computer (or even a paper diary) and delete or cross them off as you do them.
- Set up timescales and deadlines to deal with tasks.
- When you have a number of objectives at different locations, try and group tasks together so that you can achieve a cluster of objectives in the same location, and then move on.

- Avoid switching rapidly between activities: try to maintain your energy and focus despite distractions.
- Avoid getting side-tracked into other, less important and unplanned activities. Make assertive judgements about costs/benefits and be prepared to say 'no' if the balance is not in your favour.
- Ensure you have an agenda before going into meetings (what do you wish to achieve, and are the key people coming?), keep track of time during meetings, and maintain a steady flow of topics discussed and future agendas set.
- Delegate less important tasks to others who are keen to impress you: do the important things yourself to ensure that they get done well (unless you can delegate to someone very reliable) and that you don't waste time in chasing people up. Build up your delegating skills and you will find that you have more time to yourself (think about what to delegate, to whom, and how you will follow up on their progress).
- Don't be too busy to take short breaks, which allow you time to relax, reflect and regroup, as well as to plan and consult with others.
- Make people aware of your time limits – express how busy you are, as if you are late for something, and get down to business quickly, e.g.
  - 'What can I do for you?'
  - 'I really have to go.'

Ensure that the key message/questions they have are given first, so you don't end up spending time chatting idly without achieving anything.

FINANCIAL MANAGEMENT

According to the BMA Survey of Medical Students Finances in 2003–4, final-year medical students graduated with £14 903 of debt. This is now considered the norm, and it is set to get worse every year. Debt becomes a significant problem when it stops you doing important things, or when it becomes such a source of worry that it affects your concentration or health.

There are two ways of handling debt: to recognize the problem and take steps to sort it out, or to ignore it and hope things get better on their own.

When debt becomes a problem for you, as with anything, you need to form a strategy to help you deal with it. Ask yourself:

- What am I spending my money on, and is each expense necessary (form a written budget, or use a computer program such as Microsoft Money)?
- How can I save money?
- How can I increase my income ?

When you have answered these questions, write out an action plan which will contain practical steps you can follow to help you address your 'debt mountain'. Consult broadly with your friends and family – have they had similar problems? What did they do? How do they cope with the same problems?

Financial management programs such as Microsoft Money are useful in that they will allow you to graphically track how your finances are doing over time to see what effect a change you implement can have; they will also allow you to predict how things will change if you do nothing (allowing you to plan targets, and hence your future). They also provide a neat and permanent record of your finances. This prevents you losing track of your money. It sounds painful and boring, but once set up it is with you for life (in fact, it can serve as a useful reminder in later life, when you may have more disposable cash).

Practical steps for effective financial management

- Use student discounts whenever possible. For example, London Transport gives students discounts on travel cards. Other discounts include a Young Person's Rail Card, discounts on clothes (Burton) and on stationery (Partners Stationers), to name but a few.
- Get a job during those long summer holidays (medical secretarial work pays well and may provide useful experience

looking at medicine from another angle – during the first three years of medical school I made over £12 000 through such summer work – to this day I still receive the occasional call from the same agency for work).

- Remember that you won't pay any tax on your earnings if you make less than about £4500 per year (you will only pay national insurance).
- Try and apply for as much funding as possible for your intercalated BSc, elective and SSM projects – there are many prizes available which often receive few applications (in my time at medical school I was awarded over £16 000 in scholarships, prizes and awards through such applications). Plan ahead for these and gather information from your supervisor and personal tutor – they may be able to point you in the right direction.
- Try and see if you can transfer your credit card balances to a lower-rate card.
- If appropriate, express your concerns to your parents – they may be able to help.
- Your medical school has money in the form of hardship funds and hardship loans which you can apply for: enquire about these at your registry and apply as soon as possible.
- The Royal College of Surgeons of England also offers financial help to those in need via the MacLoghlin and Morris Scholarship:

  http://www.rcseng.ac.uk/surgical/research/awards/
  macloghlin_html

- Hunt around at freshers' fairs for discount cards and free merchandise.
- Break the cycle of spend now and save later by setting up a standing order (say £20 a week) from your current account to a high-interest savings account. This will ensure that you start saving straight away, and will enable you to graduate with a lump sum that you could use to buy a car, and so on. It will also provide a reservoir of emergency money should you need it earlier. Make sure you shop around for a competitive interest rate.

● Try to extend your interest-free overdraft whenever you can: the more capacity you have, the more flexibility you will have within your own financial framework.

STRESS MANAGEMENT

The key to stress management is to investigate the potential causes of your stress (the stressors) and why you have chosen to react emotionally and physically in this way (fear, anxiety, muscle tension, and so on). Once you have identified the possible causes, draw up a plan to reduce their effects. The most common causes are poor time and/or financial management (after reading the sections above, hopefully you can get started on those). Once you have reduced/minimized the 'inputs', consider your reaction.

Why are you choosing to get stressed or anxious when you receive such inputs (are they life-threatening or something?). We know that different people exposed to the same stressors will react differently. Certain personality traits have a role to play here. Do you tend to take on too much? Have you been able to draw clear boundaries between your life at medical school and your personal life? Remember, not all stress is bad: some stressors, such as competition, inspire you to achieve, so try and keep things in perspective and maintain a balance.

Practical tips for effective stress management

● Take a break, relax and do something enjoyable while thinking about the stress at the same time – can you resolve it all in your own mind?
● Try to go to bed earlier and wake up earlier: if you achieve a lot between the hours of 8am and 12pm, it can make you feel as if you're ahead of the game.
● Don't dig yourself a hole and take on more than you can handle, or raise expectations unnecessarily.
● Don't forget the importance of exercise, a balanced diet and relaxation.

- Discuss the situation with parents and friends if appropriate.
- Keep a longer-term perspective on what you are trying to achieve.
- Think about your past achievements and how much more you are capable of.
- Don't defeat yourself with stress: face up to the stressors and deal with them.
- Put the stress into context – you have on average, another 60 years to live, and you are getting stressed in your prime – is it worth it?

In their article 'Pulling the plug on stress' Cryer *et al.* (2003) discuss a five-step technique they describe as 'freeze-frame'. When you find yourself in a stressful situation or feel 'stressed':

1. Recognize and disengage – take time out from your thoughts and feelings and step back from them. This prevents the stress getting any worse.
2. Breathe through your heart – shift your focus to the area around your heart: feel your breath come in through that area and out through your solar plexus. This is thought to bring your heart rate and breathing rhythms into synchrony. The brain associates such physiological coherence with feelings of security and wellbeing.
3. Invoke a positive feeling – a walk in the park on a sunny day, or being surrounded by friends.
4. Ask yourself, is there a better alternative? – what would be an efficient, effective attitude or action that would destress your system?
5. Note the change in perspective – quietly sense any change in perception or feeling, and sustain it as long as you can.

FURTHER READING

Berglas S. Chronic time abuse. *Harvard Business Review* 2004; June: 90–7.

Cryer B, McCraty R, Childre D. Pull the plug on stress. *Harvard Business Review* 2003; July: 102–7.

3

USING INFORMATION TECHNOLOGY TO GIVE YOU AN EDGE

Mohammad Al-Ubaydli

In 1912 Dr Alexis Carrel received a Nobel Prize for his work on sewing. This included a 1908 lifesaving transfusion for a neonate that was severely anaemic after delivery. In a surgical first, he was able to suture the father's left radial artery to the baby's right popliteal vein, in a culmination of years of his experimental work on animals. Carrel pioneered this kind of delicate surgery, and invented many of the suturing techniques still in use today. To reach this level of skill he had undertaken an ambitious programme of self-training after qualifying as a surgeon in France. This began with an apprenticeship under one of Paris' finest seamstresses.

Medicine has always depended for its advances on doctors willing to train in the disciplines of other professions. This is how new technology can enter into clinical practice. Initially it seemed strange – but anyone who teased Dr Carrel for going to sewing classes was silenced in theatre, watching the delicacy of his stitches.

Computer technology can bring many benefits to medical practice. However, many clinicians are apprehensive about it because of common misunderstandings, so it is worth clearing up some myths. First, you are never too old to learn. It was my father who taught me how to use a computer, and his skills were self-taught.

Second, you do not need a degree in computer science before you are allowed to play with a computer. Unlike clinical medicine, learning on a computer allows for easy and safe experimentation.

Finally, just because you are not going to specialize in medical computing, it does not mean you cannot improve your clinical practice by learning about computers. Every doctor's early training includes some of the suturing techniques that Carrel pioneered, and a little computer knowledge can go a long way in helping your clinical education and giving you the edge over others in your career path.

HOW TO GET THE COMPUTER SKILLS YOU NEED

So, how do you begin dabbling in computers? The simplest and cheapest way is to get a book. For example, many people make use of the *Dummy's Guides* (http://www.dummies.com). Do not underestimate the educational value of this series. Each book assumes little starting knowledge but can impart a lot to the reader. If these books are not your style, there are literally hundreds of others for all levels and most tastes. One excellent book is Trefor Roscoe's *Rapid Reference To Computing in General Practice*, which is aimed at doctors. It packs a lot of advice into a pocket-sized book.

However learning from a book can be a lonely pursuit, and sometimes it is good to have a teacher setting the pace and going over the difficult concepts. A surprisingly good (and free) solution to this is the Barnes and Noble University. Barnes and Noble is the largest chain of bookstores in the USA (and the world). Its website (http://www.bn.com) has a 'University' section which runs courses continuously. You can sign up for these for free, and many of them revolve around computers (although I enjoyed the Japanese history course). The company hopes that you will buy the 'set text' from its website, but this is certainly not a requirement for the course.

At some point, you may decide that you need formal tuition. For me, it was the local polytechnic. I took a gap year before joining medical school and I enjoyed that year for the academic freedom it gave me. I was able to study exactly what I wanted, the teaching was excellent, and the students, many of them halfway through their careers, were from an excitingly diverse range of backgrounds.

Most universities and polytechnics offer the European Computer Driving Licence (http://www.ecdl.co.uk). Employers understand that the qualification indicates useful skills, and in fact the ECDL is the reference standard for the NHS (http://www.ecdl.co.uk/nhs.php?style=scn).

If you get hooked, many universities offer courses devoted to the art and science of using computers in a medical setting. The courses gently introduce health professionals to the issues involved in deploying information technology (IT), then provide a solid understanding of how to assemble solutions. The UK Health Informatics Society's website lists many of these (http://www.bmis.org/courses.html).

GET A PET

Picking up new habits is difficult. For example, after a heart attack most patients understand the importance of exercise and weight loss for their cardiovascular health. But they also find adopting these major lifestyle changes quite difficult.

One of my general practitioner mentors taught me a marvellous alternative: he advises his patients to get a pet. Whereas many people find exercise boring and difficult to maintain, exercising the dog is another matter entirely. A patient will gladly and regularly walk their dog, to the benefit of their own heart and health.

Similarly, you should consider getting a computer 'pet'. A handheld computer is a small computer that has many advantages over desktop or laptop machines. It is small and lightweight, and has a long battery life. This means you can carry it everywhere with you on your long clinical day, including lectures, libraries and wards. The machine is also fast and always switched on, and hence ready whenever you need it to be. Prices are reasonable, from £100 for a good machine.

However, the most 'pet'-like quality is that the machine is delightfully simple to use, and carries your personal data. If your past experiences with computers have been unpleasant, consider getting a handheld computer. Visit www.handheldsfordoctors.com/learn for more information and clinical reviews on how to get you started.

HOW TO USE IT TO GIVE YOURSELF AN EDGE

Information technology can help at various stages in your medical career. For example, you can use a spreadsheet program for the collection and analysis of your research data, a word processing program for writing a paper or book about your data and a presentation program to create a slide show for talking about your paper at conferences. A word processing program is also essential for writing your CV, and many students write their lecture notes using word processing or presentation software.

This section focuses on the most common programs – Microsoft Word (word processor), Microsoft Excel (spreadsheet) – and Microsoft PowerPoint (presentation program) is discussed in Chapter 11. There are plenty of alternative software packages out there, including Open Office, which is free (http://www.openoffice.org) and includes all these software tools and more.

Tips for Microsoft Word – word processing software

Word's outliner is the key to the kingdom. It is analogous to classifying your medical lists, because it gives structure to your content and order to your presentation, but it takes a little discipline.

Select Outline from the View menu. Then, start writing. The letters are large: you are writing the title of your document, known as a Level 1 heading. You will also notice a new set of icons under the menu (Figure 3.1).

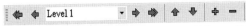

Fig. 3.1 The outliner toolbar. Reproduced courtesy of Microsoft Word.

Start a new line, click the ➡ icon and write some more text. The letters are slightly smaller, because you are writing a Level 2 heading. This is because you have demoted it into a subheading of the Level 1 heading. Clicking the ⬅ icon reverses this. There are nine levels of heading, and if you press the ⇨ icon the text becomes Body text, which is the level for normal paragraph text. Using these three icons, you can structure your entire document.

Add some styles

The outliner also controls the presentation of your text. From the Format menu, select Styles and Formatting. Click on Heading 2, for example, and choose Modify. You can use this to change any aspect of Level 2 headings, including the typeface, the size and the line spacing. Word then applies this change to all the text that is Level 2.

Themes are even better. From the Format menu select Theme, and choose from the list of available themes. Word instantly applies your choice to all text at all levels.

Track your changes

When you are happy with your draft, send it to colleagues for review. From the File menu, choose Send To then Mail Recipient (As Attachment). Word will use your email software to send an email to your colleagues with your document attached.

Most importantly, in the email that you write, ask your colleagues to choose Track Changes from the Tools menu when they open the attached document. When they eventually email the file back to you, much of the text will be red. Word will have kept track of the reviewer's deletions, insertions and substitutions. Move the mouse over this text and click the *right* mouse button: a menu appears offering you the choice of accepting or rejecting the change you clicked on. Go through the whole text in this way and you will have a structured, well presented and correct document.

Tips for Adobe PDF

The ability of word processors to track your changes to a document is useful, but also dangerous. For example, one job applicant sent me their CV in Microsoft Word format. I could see all the changes they had made to their CV (some of them quite amateurish) and the comments from earlier reviewers (some of them quite damning). Never send your CV to anyone as a word-processed document.

Even the basic ability of word processing software to edit text is a danger. For example, many teachers prepare notes about their lectures and email them to their students. This saves effort, time and paper. The problem arises when one of the students edits the document and shares it with others. Consider what would happen if a student accidentally deleted the decimal point for a recommended drug dosage, and then sent it to others with your name as the author of the document. Never send a completed word-processed document electronically.

Instead, you should send such documents in portable document format (PDF). This was originally developed by Adobe to allow the creation of documents that appear the same on any computer. This was important for conference organizers, for example, who had found that their carefully laid-out posters could lose their arrangement when viewed on different computer screens. PDF documents also have the advantage of hiding their review history, and making further editing of the document difficult (but attributable).

Converting your word processed document to PDF format is easy using Open Office. From the 'File' menu, select 'Export as PDF. . . '. The software will ask you to name the PDF file, and will then create it. You can safely email this file to colleagues.

If you are using Microsoft Word, or another word processor, then the easiest and cheapest solution is PDF995 (http://www.pdf995.com). The software creates PDF files, and costs $9.95. The trial is free, however, so all you have to do to get started is download and install the software. It will add a virtual printer to your computer. To convert your word-processed document to PDF, select 'Print. . .' from the 'File' menu. Next, select 'PDF995' as your printer, and type in the name of the PDF file. Again, you can safely email this file to colleagues.

To open the file, you and your colleagues will need Adobe Reader. This is available free of charge from http://www.acrobat.com, and works on most computers, including Windows PCs and Macs. In fact, you almost certainly already have the software, as most computer manufacturers include it.

Tips for Microsoft Excel – spreadsheet software

Microsoft Excel can store tables of your data, and then perform calculations within those tables. A new document begins as an empty table. Click on the area of the table where you would like to add data, and type it in.

To add up all the cells in a column, click inside the cell where you want the sum to appear. Type in = SUM(. Keep the shift key pressed and click inside the first cell in the column. Then type a : (colon) mark. With the shift key still pressed, click at the bottom of the column. Finally, close the brackets by typing), and press the return key.

The sum of the column will appear, and this is an example of a formula in action. Excel provides many other formulae, including statistical tools such as the mean and standard deviation. To use these, click the f_x button, and Excel will take you through the steps.

You can also create graphs from your data. Click in the top left-hand corner of your table. With the shift key pressed, click in the bottom right corner. Press the F11 key and Excel creates a chart for you. To override its choices, click twice. For example, to change the typeface of the x-axis, click twice on the axis, click Font and choose your font.

Of course, all these tools depend on good and comprehensive datas collecting, which requires a lot of time. Furthermore, in a busy hospital environment, getting access to the notes for an audit project can be a haphazard and temporary affair. Always carry a handheld computer. Most Palm Powered handheld computers come with ExcelToGo, whereas Pocket PC handheld computers come with Pocket Excel. Data you enter there will easily transfer to your desktop computer's Microsoft Excel.

TIPS ON SEARCHING THE INTERNET

The Internet is an enormous library, likely to contain the information that you need. Getting to that information can be difficult, however, but some websites specialize in helping you with the search. These are called 'search engines' and there are two types: general ones such as Google, and clinical ones such as PubMed.

Google and other general search engines

By far the most popular search engine is Google (http://www.google.com). This earned its popularity because of its power and simplicity. A more recent tool is Teoma (http://www.teoma.com), which provides even better results but is not as well known. The tips in this section work with either search engine.

Open your computer's web browser and type 'www.google.com' in the address bar at the top. Press the Go button, and you will see something like Figure 3.2. A 'query' is the text that you must type into a search engine (your question), and a 'results page' is the list that the engine produces (its answer).

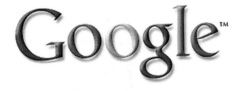

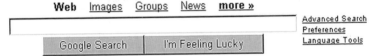

Fig. 3.2 www.google.com.

The more specific your query, the more helpful the results page. For example, if you are searching for the success rates of hip replacements in the UK, your query should not be 'hip replacements'. Try 'hip replacements success' instead. Figure 3.3 shows the results page.

For a website to be included in the results page it must contain words that were part of your query. To ensure that the site was written by doctors, use medical words. Try 'hip replacements efficacy'.

You can also restrict the search engine's answers to a certain set of pages by adding 'site:' at the end of your query. For NHS sites, try 'hip replacements efficacy site:nhs.uk'. For a paper on a Cambridge University Professor's website, try 'hip replacements efficacy site:cam.ac.uk'.

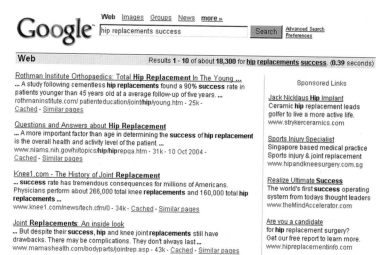

Fig. 3.3 Google results page.

The results page includes a link labelled 'images'. To see pictures of hip prostheses try 'hip prosthesis', then click 'images'. This is extremely useful for PowerPoint presentations. Finally, note that most search engines only accept the first 10 words of your query. Choose these carefully. For these and other tips, consider carrying the excellent *Google Pocket Guide* in your bag.

Pubmed

To find clinical literature, use the PubMed search engine (http://www.pubmed.gov). This has abstracts of much of the modern biomedical literature. If someone has done an experiment that gives an answer to your question, you will probably find the abstract of the paper on PubMed. However, to navigate this huge amount of information you need to learn a few tricks. For example, consider how to use PubMed to find out the percentage of stroke patients that develop epilepsy.

Open your web browser and type 'www.pubmed.gov' in the address bar. Press the Go button, and you will see something like Figure 3.4. In the top right-hand corner is the logo of the

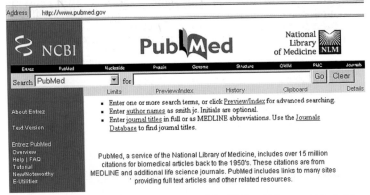

Fig. 3.4 PubMed. Reproduced courtesy of the National Library of Medicine.

United States National Library of Medicine (NLM), which runs the website. The top left corner shows the logo of the NLM's National Center for Biotechnology Information (NCBI). The NCBI has databases on gene sequences, proteins, entire textbooks, and of course PubMed.

The website helpfully defaults to 'Search PubMed for' something, a little below the logos. That 'something' is your query. For example, if you type in 'stroke patients with epilepsy' and click the Go button, the website would search the database for that phrase. As you can see from the results page, however, 'stroke patients with epilepsy' is a bad phrase for PubMed. At the time of writing PubMed found matching 645 papers, most of which are not quite what we had in mind: it is not specific enough. PubMed searches for whatever you ask it to. The answer you are looking for will probably be in those 645 papers, but being specific gets you the right answer quickly.

There are several ways to refine the question. First, we asked about 'stroke'. Did we mean 'cerebrovascular accident', or did we mean the verb 'to stroke'? Second, did we want papers that were about strokes, or papers that mentioned the word stroke somewhere in them? Third, we mentioned 'patients with

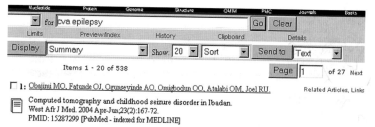

Fig. 3.5 Search results. Reproduced courtesy of the National Library of Medicine.

epilepsy'. Did we want data from trials counting the percentage of patients who went on to develop epilepsy, or did we want anecdotal case reports where a stroke patient developed epilepsy?

Let's start with stroke. You should use CVA instead. And because epilepsy is unambiguous, you can type 'cva epilepsy'.

At the time of writing, pressing the Go button showed 538 papers in the results page (Figure 3.5). It is a little easier to go through these, but there is one more trick. Click on 'limits', just under the text of the question. This takes you to a page that allows you to narrow down your question in all sorts of ways (Figure 3.6). In this case, you want to make sure that your answer comes from a trial. Click on 'Publication Types' and

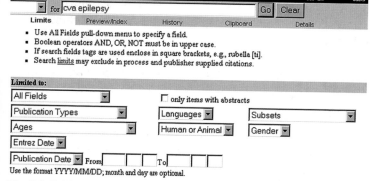

Fig. 3.6 PubMed limits page. Reproduced courtesy of the National Library of Medicine.

choose 'Randomized Controlled Trial'. Then click the 'Go' button. At the time of writing this produced just one paper, and its title was 'Incidence and predictors for post-stroke epilepsy.' Click on the title to read the abstract (Figure 3.7).

☐1: Intern Med J. 2004 May;34(5):243-9.

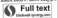

Neurological manifestations of cardiac myxoma: a review of the literature and report of cases.

Ekinci EI, Donnan GA.

Austin and Repatriation Medical Centre, Melbourne, Victoria, Australia. eekinci2002@yahoo.com.au

BACKGROUND AND AIMS: Cardiac myxoma is a rare but important cause of stroke, which affects young people. More recently the diagnosis has been enhanced by the use of echocardiograms. We aimed to review the neurological presentations, including stroke, of cardiac myxoma in this modern era of diagnosis and management. METHODS: Records of patients with neurological presentations at the Austin and Repatriation Medical Centre and The Northern Hospital were retrieved from 1985 to late 2001, using International Classification of Diseases codes for atrial myxoma. Published literature reports were obtained by using Medline search database. An iterative process of bibliography review was utilised to identify reports not found by primary search. Case demographics, neurological presentations, investigations, treatment and outcome were recorded. RESULTS: From the Austin and Repatriation Medical Centre and The Northern Hospital, 6 cases were reported in detail and 107 cases from the published literature were analysed. The mean age of all cases was 43 (range 6-82). There was a female to male predominance (3:2). While there were overlapping neurological presentations, the most common presentation was ischaemic stroke (83% of all patients) most often in multiple sites (41%). The other presentations included syncope (28%), psychiatric presentations (23%), headache (15%) and seizures (12%). Commonest means of reaching the diagnosis was by echocardiography. The myxoma was surgically resected in 69% of cases. Of all cases, 24% were autopsy reports, almost all prior to availability of echocardiograms (in mid-1970s). CONCLUSIONS: Patients who presented with neurological complications of cardiac myxoma were young and stroke was by far the most common single presentation. Importantly, when all clinical manifestations were considered, almost half were potentially reversible. In recent years, echocardiography has made significant contribution to establishing the diagnosis less invasively. There is uncertainty about the role of anticoagulants. The treatment of choice remains surgical excision, although the timing post stroke is debatable. There is a need for large scale collaborative studies to help refine management strategies.

Publication Types:
• Review
• Review of Reported Cases

PMID: 15151670 [PubMed - indexed for MEDLINE]

Fig. 3.7 Abstract of Lossius MI *et al.* Incidence and predictors for post-stroke epilepsy. A prospective controlled trial. The Akershus stroke study. *Eur J Neurol* 2002; 9(4):365–8. Reproduced courtesy of the National Library of Medicine.

It contains the sentence 'Twelve patients (2.5%) developed PSE [post-stroke epilepsy] during 12 months', which is a good start. But of course you should read the full paper to understand all the caveats. For example, the study involves a small number of patients and you would need to know the error margins for the study. The *British Medical Journal* (BMJ) has an excellent guide on this called 'How to read a paper' (http://bmj.bmjjournals.com/collections/read.shtml).

To read the full paper, click the 'Full text' button. PubMed provides these buttons to take you to the paper on the publisher's website. Every publisher has different pricing policies, but if the journal is well established, and you are using a computer in your medical school's library, the chances are that you will be able to read the full paper because your school will have already paid the journal's publisher.

Finally, PubMed has many more features that should support you in answering questions throughout your medical career. On the left-hand side of the page you will see the links 'Help' and 'Tutorial'. The first one gives you a clear explanation of every feature, and clicking the 'Tutorial' link gives you a guided tour.

This brings me to the end of this guided tour of medical computing. I hope that you put these tools to use at medical school and in your subsequent clinical practice, and I wish you joy in your future learning.

FURTHER READING

Calishain T, Dornfest R, Adams DJ. *Google Pocket Guide*, 1st edn. Farnham: O'Reilly, 2003.
http://www.handheldsfordoctors.com/book/text/chapter2.htm
Roscoe, T. *Rapid Reference to Computing in General Practice*. London: Mosby, 2003.

4

HOW TO FIND INFORMATION IN MEDICINE

Martin Hewitt

Medicine as a profession is extremely reliant on information. In recognition of this, the NHS has launched some major information initiatives: the National Knowledge Service, the National Library for Health, the NHS Institute for Learning, Skills and Innovation and the National Programme for Information Technology in the NHS are just some of the more recent developments.

In their day to day work, doctors may consult electronic patient records, research articles, web discussion forums, email, patients, pharmaceutical industry advertisements and many other sources. The ability to handle information is fundamental to your career as a student and as a doctor:

- Information for your coursework, research projects and SSMs.
- Clinical decision making: which treatment is most appropriate? How do you find out?
- Keeping up with new research, clinical developments, government policy and so on.
- Maintaining these skills after graduation for continuing professional development.

When you leave university, your knowledge base is likely to go into rapid decline unless you develop good information management skills. Information is being produced in unprecedented quantities. Without these skills, you risk being overwhelmed, unable to find the really useful facts and ideas you need, and end up being information averse. A great deal of information is out there, but not all of it is reliable. This is a problem for everyone, but in clinical practice the quality of information can be literally a matter of life and death. So where do you start?

BOOKS

Always start with textbooks. They usually contain a good overview of a subject area and are essential when you are learning something from scratch. Your tutors will give you lists of recommended books, but read more widely to gain a deeper understanding. Books are still mainly available in print, but an increasing number are now available online.

Use your college's library catalogue to find books. Library or information service staff will be able to advise you on how to use it. Textbooks are usually quite general. If you were looking for information about treating circulatory disorders in people with diabetes, try searching for general books about diabetes, rather than a whole book on this specific question.

The drawback with books is the time lag between writing and publication, which may be years. For subjects where the state of knowledge is not developing very rapidly, this is not a big problem, but if you need to know about the latest drug treatments for a particular condition, you may well find that textbooks are less useful.

JOURNALS

Journals are much more current. They are the most important means of disseminating biomedical research findings and keeping up with new developments. Many research journals are now available on the Internet, with archives usually going back to the mid-1990s, although there are initiatives under way to make older material available online as well. Older material may be available in print in your college library.

Access to electronic journals can be confusing. Your college will subscribe to a range of journals from different publishers. Each publisher has its own requirements: some need passwords, others check your computer's address; a few are freely available. Most journals offer an archive of previous issues and a basic search facility. If you know which paper you want, use the archive or browse option to locate it. If you don't know of a specific paper on your subject, use a database such as Medline first (see below).

When you find the paper you want, you will probably see a number of options: a link to an abstract, a link to 'full text' or 'HTML' and a link to 'PDF'. What do these mean?

- Abstract – a short summary of the paper. Use this to decide its relevance.
- Full text or HTML – the full text, displayed as a web page. This is useful if you want to scan it by eye but don't want to keep a copy. You can use all the familiar features of the web: you can follow links, you can enlarge graphics and so on.
- PDF – portable document format. This displays the paper just as it appears in print. This is usually easier to read and better for printing, but you lose the advantages of HTML. To view PDFs, use Adobe Acrobat, which you can obtain free from http://www.adobe.com; other pdf readers are also available.

If your paper is not available on the web, check your college library catalogue to see whether you have access to the print version of the journal. If not, ask about interlibrary loan facilities or access to other institutions' libraries, including the British Library.

Your tutors may recommend particular papers, but eventually you will want to find papers yourself. The best way to do this is to use an online bibliographic database.

MEDLINE AND OTHER DATABASES

To find papers on your subject, use a bibliographic database. You can carry out simple or complicated searches and limit what you find by publication year, age group and many other criteria. You can usually save your results, email them to yourself, or simply print them.

The best-known biomedical database is Medline. It covers clinical medicine and biomedical research, but also includes dentistry, pharmacology, microbiology, nutrition and psychiatry. It's important to be able to search effectively, so ask your library or information service about training.

Get to know Medline first. Medline is not comprehensive, though, so when you feel comfortable using it, have a look at some others, for example:

- **Embase:** this has similar coverage to Medline, with more extensive coverage of European literature. It includes pharmacy, pharmacology, toxicology, public health, psychiatry and forensic science. It is particularly useful for drug information.
- **PsycINFO:** a major psychology resource. It also covers psychiatry, education, medicine, nursing and social work.
- **Web of Knowledge:** access to **Science Citation Index** and **Social Sciences Citation Index**. Science Citation Index includes biomedical sciences, clinical medicine, dentistry and health sciences.
- **CINAHL:** the major database for nursing and allied health.

It helps to know how databases work. The producers create a record for each paper they index, containing all the information that you need to locate the paper. This information is put into different *fields* in the record: e.g. the author field, title field, and so on. You can search for information in one or more of these fields.

Computers are very literal. If you search for *cancer* in the title, you will retrieve exactly that: papers with the word 'cancer' appearing in the title. You won't see papers where the author has used a term such as *carcinoma* or *tumour*, or even *cancers*. Different authors often vary considerably in the kind of terminology they use to discuss the same subject.

Many databases address this problem by using subject headings. Although different authors might use a variety of terms to discuss cancer, the database indexers will give all the general papers about cancer a single subject heading: in Medline, this is *neoplasms*. If we search for this subject heading we can retrieve all those general papers, instead of having to search for all the variant terms that might have been used.

Medline's subject headings are known as the Medical Subject Headings (MeSH). These are also used to index books in many medical school libraries and in online resources such as OMNI. You can use the MeSH via Medline to identify key terminology in your subject. You can often improve the results of web searches by using these terms.

Many databases offer direct links to the full text of papers or the ability to transfer records to reference management software (see below).

You should create a list of the references you have found:

● To locate paper versions using your local library catalogue when you cannot access the full article online.
● So you can cite them correctly (see below).

Your medical school library or information service will have subscribed to a number of databases, provided by a variety of commercial publishers. Each publisher uses their own *interface*: i.e. the features you use to search the database. You will probably find that you encounter more than one interface, such as Dialog or Ovid. Remember, though, that the actual information content of the database will be the same regardless of interface.

Most databases are only available via subscription, but Medline is also freely available on the web via PubMed. This includes a variety of useful features and it's worth getting to know how to use it. Medline is published by the US National Library of Medicine, who provide a wide range of other very useful information resources for anyone involved in health care. Their website can be found at http://www.nlm.nih.gov.

THE INTERNET

There are two pervasive myths about the web:

- If it's not on Google, it's not on the web.
- If it's not on the web, it doesn't exist.

Neither is true.

Many people at university feel confident about using the Internet. Most of us search the web frequently and usually find general information quite readily. Most of us are also familiar with the many frustrations of web searching. Look up *Prozac* on Google. In less than a second, you will get a list of over 2 million links. This will include some very useful information, but there will also be sites trying to make money out of the unwary, misleading sites, campaigning websites, as well as information you can rely on in your work. Who would wade through all 2 million records anyway?

Never start with a search engine when you look for health information. Use the National Library for Health: http://www.library.nhs.uk, a single point of access to many major resources for health practitioners, including:

- Access to important databases.
- Specialist libraries covering information for specific areas of health care.

- A clinical guidelines finder.
- Access to National Services Frameworks, care pathways and clinical protocols.

If you don't find what you want, try these routes:

- Use sites produced by trusted organizations. Start with your college's library or information services pages.
- Do you already know some good sites? They may link to other good sites.
- Evaluated subject gateways contain lists of web resources which have been assessed for quality and reliability. There are some very good medical gateways, including OMNI, BIOME and Healthfinder.

For information on other subjects, try the Resource Discovery Network (RDN): http://www.rdn.ac.uk. The RDN also contains Internet Medic, a tutorial about assessing quality on the web.

Ask yourself these questions:

- **Who** produced it? Is the organization one you already know and trust? Is the author of the document you're looking at qualified? Is there an *About Us* page? If not, ask yourself why not?
- **Evidence.** Is there evidence for the claims being made? What is the quality of that evidence? Does it reference key statements and point to the existing literature?
- **Content.** Is it up to date? When was the page last updated? Are there many broken links?
- **Relevance.** Is this site intended for you? In what country is it published? Does the local context affect its relevance?
- **Miracles.** Talk of miracle cures and 'amazing results' is always *very* suspicious.

When you use search engines, improve your chances of finding reliable information by:

- Using the **advanced search** options. Use the online help pages to guide you.
- Using **technical or professional terminology** to focus your search.

Don't restrict yourself to one search engine. None is comprehensive, and they all work differently.

OTHER SOURCES

Everything you need is not necessarily on the web. Here are some other sources:

- **Reports of biomedical meetings and conferences.**
- **Reference books:** dictionaries, encyclopaedias and so on.
- **Theses and dissertations:** you can often find cutting-edge ideas here which would never find their way into a book or journal.
- **Official publications and statistics:** reports from government agencies, government white papers, scientific associations, international organizations, surveys, guidelines, legislation, regulations, and so on.
- **People:** students, academics, clinicians and patients are all unique and valuable sources of information and guidance.

EVIDENCE-BASED PRACTICE

Evidence-based practice (EBP) is an approach which argues that clinical interventions should be based on a combination of the best available external evidence as to their effectiveness, clinicians' own expertise and experience, and the patient's or population's unique needs and preferences. It has been widely adopted.

There are a number of EBP resources. Many are available via the National Library for Health:

- The **Cochrane Library** includes full text systematic reviews and references to controlled trials.
- **Clinical Evidence** summarizes the current state of knowledge and uncertainty about the prevention and treatment of clinical conditions. It provides guidance on putting evidence into practice.

- The TriP (Turning Research into Practice) Database searches many EBP websites in one go. If your college subscribes, you will have access to advanced features. If not, use the more basic version.

Other EBP resources may be listed on your college website, or try King's College London's EBP page (http://www.kcl.ac.uk/depsta/iss/schools/bdhmn/subjsources/ebp/ebp.html) or *Netting the Evidence* at the University of Sheffield.

ACKNOWLEDGING YOUR SOURCES

When you use the information you find in an essay or another piece of work, always acknowledge your source. Presenting someone else's ideas as your own is plagiarism, so always make it clear when you are quoting someone else, and include a reference to the source (print or electronic) in a bibliography at the end of your work. There are conventions for how to do this: check your own college's requirements and guidelines.

KEEPING TRACK

To make it easier, keep a note of everything you find and where you found it. Some students use reference management software, such as Reference Manager, EndNote, or the simpler versions of RefWorks or WriteNote. These are software packages you can use to organize your references and find them easily again. The software will renumber the reference both in the text and in your bibliography section as well. Your references are stored for the next time you do a project on the same subject, ready to be inserted whenever you want at the touch of a button.

These programs can save you a huge amount of time. It's worth learning how to use them once you start regularly consulting databases and other resources for your coursework. You are likely to use them throughout your career whenever you write scientific papers, case reports, or publish trials or reports. You may be able to pick them up at a discount through your university library or information service. Ask if they offer training on how to use them as well.

OVERVIEW

- A vast amount of information is available. Good information retrieval and management skills are essential for all medics.
- Start with textbooks. Use your college's library catalogue to find them.
- Use research journals for more current information and more specialized research. Use your college's library catalogue to find them. To find out what has been published, use bibliographic databases.
- Bibliographic databases such as Medline contain references to journal papers.
- The web: use search engines as a last resort. Always consider the quality of what you find.
- There are many other sources of information, including official publications, reference tools and so on.
- Evidence-based practice: it's important to become familiar with what it's about and the sources of information specifically designed for EBP.
- Always acknowledge your sources and include a bibliography at the end of anything you hand in for assessment.

King's College London's web pages includes access to, and advice on, all of the above and more: http://www.kcl.ac.uk/iss.

PART

II

MAKING THE BIG DECISIONS AT MEDICAL SCHOOL

5

INTERCALATED DEGREES – BENEFITS, COSTS AND ALTERNATIVES

Riaz Agha

INTRODUCTION

An intercalated degree is an extra year's study, usually inserted between the second and third years of the medical course, with the aim of studying a subject at greater depth and gaining a BSc, BA or BMedSci degree. Studying for an intercalated degree is becoming increasingly popular, with about 30–40 per cent of UK medical students opting for them in 1998. Although the proportion varies between medical schools, this figure is likely to have risen, with an intercalated degree being made compulsory at, among others, University College London and Imperial College of Medicine. Furthermore, the number of medical graduates with a BSc, BA or BMedSci degree is increasing with the formation of graduate 'fast-track' 4-year degree programmes (e.g. at St George's Medical School, London).

Although some medical schools have made intercalated degrees compulsory, some have reserved them only for those that score the highest marks in the previous years (e.g. Leicester), and still others give students an open choice provided that they pass the previous year's exams at the first attempt (GKT – Guy's, King's and St Thomas' medical schools).

The decision as to whether to do an intercalated degree is one of the most important that you as a medical student can make, but it is far from straightforward. It is an individual cost-benefit calculation that has long-term consequences. The key requirement of the decision-maker is having the information available to assess the costs, the benefits and alternatives. You can then go about making the right decision for you and your career.

POTENTIAL BENEFITS

Personal development

Doing an intercalated degree is very different from the first two years of the course. Many of the exams and assessments are essay rather than multiple-choice question-based. This will teach you to think more creatively and to construct logical arguments in a scientific manner for and against different theoretical positions. This scientific training is a common feature of intercalated degrees and will remain with you for life. You will improve your critical analysis skills when assessing scientific papers, improve your presentation skills, perform statistical analysis, and gain mastery of Medline and other research databases that you will use for the rest of your career, as well as a potentially greater computer literacy.

You will also learn how to conduct literature reviews, write formal essays, to take more focused lecture notes, to work independently, and to motivate yourself to accomplish set goals through self-directed learning (there is also less virtual campus support during a BSc, and attendance is a more important factor). The teaching will often be in relatively small groups compared with medicine, and you may find yourself asking more questions and thinking as an individual a lot more. It is worth noting that the workload and balance between lectures/tutorials and private study is highly variable among the different intercalated programmes.

Many students comment on how their intercalated degree changed the way they think and how it provided them with lifelong skills. In essence, a whole range of generic skills and attitudes can be picked up during the course of an intercalated degree, some of which you might not otherwise be exposed to as forcefully in the medical course. Many of these skills will be transferable and may help in the development of future parallel careers (careers in other industries or in the private sector, in addition to your main NHS career), or if you choose to leave medicine altogether.

Career development

Evered *et al.* (1987) found that those who gained research training or experience as undergraduates raised substantially more research grants and had better publication records (and were cited more often) than those without an intercalated degree. The career patterns of those who do intercalated degrees are more likely to proceed along an academic or hospital-based route, although not invariably so. The content of the degree and the options available can also have an impact on this pattern. Eaton (1985) did a retrospective study of graduates and concluded that those who did an intercalated degree were more likely to obtain honours in their medical degree, hold academic positions and subsequently publish than were a set of controls who did not intercalate.

If you are considering a career in academic medicine, the intercalated degree will provide an excellent opportunity for you to assess whether you are suitable; furthermore, all branches of academic medicine require a higher degree. In addition, certain clinical specialties, such as neurology, and some surgical specialties, expect you to have a higher degree (to which the intercalated degree is a springboard, although it is not mandatory). The intercalated degree can also help to guide future career decisions by exposing you to the basic science aspects of a particular clinical specialty.

If you do a clinical-based intercalated degree you will also have the opportunity to sample a particular specialty and assess your interest in pursuing that specialty as a career. The intercalated degree also opens up opportunities to pursue other professions (many of which don't require a specific degree) and provides an exit strategy for those who no longer wish to pursue a career in medicine. In a survey of 138 second-year medical students, 5.8 per cent stated that this was a reason for their wanting to do an intercalated degree.

Future job applications

Doing an intercalated degree can also improve a medical student's rank order position when applying for pre-registration house officer (PRHO) posts through the GKT Matching Scheme. However, many students now look beyond the PRHO year and wonder whether an intercalated degree will improve their chances of getting a senior house officer (SHO) or specialist registrar (SpR) post in the future. In fact, 81.2 per cent of medical students wanting to intercalate believe that this will improve their chances of success when applying for SHO or SpR posts, compared with only 45.7 per cent who thought that it would improve their PRHO ranking.

Students are also worried about having their CV separated into a 'have-BSc' and a 'don't have BSc' pile when it comes to shortlisting applicants for interviews. In essence, it helps both sets of applications, but simply doing an intercalated degree and getting a 2:1 (which the majority of students do) is very different from doing an intercalated degree, getting a first, plus publications and presentations on top as a byproduct of the research or essays completed as part of the course (that research project and those essays take on a different significance now – if you enter your intercalated degree with this attitude and form a good partnership with your supervisor, then the 'sky's the limit') . It is worth noting that for intercalated medical students at GKT 23.4 per cent get a first, 68.5 per cent get a 2:1, 7.5 per cent get a 2:2 and 0.64 per cent get a third – that's a one in four chance of getting a first!

With the Royal College of Surgeons of England reporting as many as 200 candidates applying for each job at SHO and SpR grades doing an intercalated degree may also be particularly advantageous for those considering a career in the more competitive medical or surgical specialties. The London Deanery's generic person specification states that having an intercalated degree is desirable for various SHO and SpR posts. Much of the literature also states that a successful intercalated degree can give you an edge when applying for jobs.

In 1999, Galasko and Smith reported the ratio of eligible basic surgical trainees (BST) to specialist registrar programmes. Over the period 1999–2002 the ratios for each specialty vary, but generally the level of competition increases. In 2002, the number of eligible BSTs to SpR places for A&E was 1:1, for urology it was 5:1, for plastic surgery it was 13:1 and for neurosurgery it was 117:0. This illustrates the level of competition in different fields, and how it can vary from year to year.

Publishing papers

The intensely competitive nature of medicine as a career has perpetuated the 'publish or perish' maxim in the minds of would-be applicants. Chambler *et al.* in 1998, in a survey of 100 postgraduate deans and regional advisers of the Royal Colleges, showed that having publications ranked second in a list of important features on a CV, with referees being ranked number one. The number of publications can often be a major differentiating criterion at SpR post interviews. An intercalated degree is also associated with a better publication record (publishing more frequently and being cited more often) relative to those who don't intercalate. Publishing a paper is also considered highly desirable for SHO and SpR job applications.

One of the best – albeit informal – indicators of the importance of publishing is the degree of coverage this issue is given in *BMJ Classified*, a journal aimed essentially at SHOs trying to secure an SpR post. Regular articles on 'how to maximize your chances to publish as a trainee', 'publish and prosper', 'publications and your other professional activities' are printed here, and many provide useful information and advice. Of course, to see your own work in print will also give you a tremendous sense of satisfaction. One article even describes publications as the Holy Grail for SHOs. Furthermore, a publication will raise your profile in certain circles and will provide material for discussion with key individuals (as well as an excuse to approach them in the first place).

Presentations at meetings

Presenting research orally or as a poster at local, regional, national or international meetings is a desirable criterion for those applying for SHO and SpR posts. It is ranked fourth in the aforementioned survey and increases your chances of being shortlisted for jobs. A presentation at an international meeting can often lead to the publication of an abstract, which will strengthen the publications section of your CV. You will also raise your profile and potentially make a variety of connections with other international researchers, who may take you on for future projects or even during your elective (incidentally, you will also have a much greater chance of being funded for a research elective if their name is on your research proposal: this requires longer-term planning and thus necessitates personal connections to be built up and strengthened over time).

Research experience

An intercalated degree that includes a research project will provide you with a whole range of skills and experiences that you may not be exposed to during the standard medical course. These include formulating a hypothesis, understanding interfering variables, asking the right questions and devising experiments to address them, statistical analysis, and drawing conclusions from the work you have done. You will also be taught – and will indeed execute – many of the experimental techniques used worldwide in relation to the research you are doing. This will teach you technical discipline and give you a greater understanding of how biological processes can be manipulated as you hover at the 'cutting edge' of science, where an open mind and the ability to 'think outside the box' is essential for success. This contrasts with the standard medical course, where much of the information is taken on trust and the opportunity to question stated 'facts' does not arise to the same degree.

You will also develop your creative abilities, not only in the design of your project but also in directing the thrust of your research based on a logical analysis of the results. It won't simply be rote learning and memorizing, as in much of years 1 and 2, of course – you need to engage in truly critical and reflective thinking, incorporating creative flair, mathematical logic and an understanding of your own limitations.

The research project is an ideal opportunity to develop relationships with a whole new set of people, including your supervisor, other scientists and the laboratory technicians. This will provide a reservoir of scientific relationships and possibly the start of a long-standing collaboration, which could provide dividends throughout the rest of your career, including future research project opportunities, advice on other research opportunities and support when applying for grants, as well as references. It is worth noting that programme advisers understandably give higher priority in allocating projects to students who are specializing in their particular programme (e.g. anatomy projects going to those doing an intercalated degree in anatomy).

Having a scientific thesis, publications and presentations under your belt indicates a continuing clinical and experimental curiosity, which could aid future job applications. This can also have implications for an elective application to a research facility, as well as your chances of scooping many of the awards and prizes available for electives. You can also extend a project into the 4 months of summer holidays you have at the end of your intercalated degree, as well as future special study modules (SSMs) (by self-designing them such that you can continue your work on your project). The Wellcome Trust funds some summer projects, so you could earn money while you continue your research (see Appendix 1).

DEVELOPMENT OF CRITICAL ANALYSIS AND EVIDENCE-BASED MEDICINE SKILLS

The modern clinician is expected to apply the principles of evidence-based medicine (EBM) to their clinical practice and decision-making. The principles of EBM are that:

- Clinicians should regularly raise structured questions about diagnosis, prognosis, therapy and so on in their encounters with patients.
- They should search systematically for research-based evidence.
- They should evaluate critically the evidence they find, asking about validity ('can I trust it?') and relevance ('does it apply to this patient?').
- They should base their clinical decisions and the information they share with patients on 'bottom-line' mathematical estimates of benefit and harm (Professor Trish Greenhalgh, 2003).

The need for students to acquire critical appraisal skills to allow them to cope with the expanding literature has never been greater. I recently suggested that the way to ensure that lifelong clinical performance incorporates the principles of

EBM is to introduce students to the practical realities of research during their formative years. This original hypothesis has been supported by others involved in medical education and curriculum development.

Doing an intercalated degree may provide you with key skills which could improve your analytical abilities for the purposes of EBM. It is important to bear in mind that the practice of EBM is not a 'behaviour': it is an internalized spirit of enquiry born out of a deep understanding of both the value and the limitations of biomedical research.

McManus *et al.* (1999) showed that students who undertake intercalated degrees have higher deep and strategic learning scores than those who do not, although there was no difference between them on entry to medical school. Furthermore, they showed a greater interest in a medical research-based career. Critical analysis skills will allow you to resolve conflicts and bias in the literature by assessing the objectives, design, methodology, results and statistics that have been utilized by different studies to obtain conflicting results and hence draw opposing conclusions. This may also lead to higher-quality research, and those who do intercalated degrees tend to have a better publication record and are cited more often, possibly as a result of these newly acquired analytical abilities.

Intellectual curiosity

About 53–72 per cent of students list broadening their knowledge, a chance to pursue a subject of interest and intellectual curiosity as some of their reasons for doing an intercalated degree. You have the unique opportunity to select the course and the units you are most interested in; this is very different from the rest of the medical course, where you may feel you are on a 'treadmill' (just running to stand still, and unable to move sideways). This intellectual freedom can be greatly rewarding, and allows you ample time to think deeply about your learning and ask questions.

OTHER ADVANTAGES

Other possible reasons for wanting to do an intercalated degree include:

- The acquisition of key skills (statistics, laboratory skills, dissection skills, etc.).
- A break from medicine.
- To stay with your friends.
- To have more time off during term-time for the pursuit of extracurricular activities.
- To have another long summer break (about four months, compared with three weeks at the end of the third year).
- You may not feel ready for clinics.
- More private study time.
- To get an extra degree in one year (or two in six years, instead of one in five).
- As a safety option/exit strategy in case something goes wrong in the clinical years.
- To meet new people (final-year BSc students and other healthcare professionals).
- To remain a student for longer.
- To approach clinical medicine in a more mature way.
- To intercalate at another university and experience life in another part of the country.
- To study a subject you may not have the opportunity to pursue later (e.g. the arts).

POTENTIAL DRAWBACKS

Unnecessary

An intercalated degree is not mandatory for getting a job, and in some careers, for example general practice, the competition is relatively low compared with hospital medicine, owing to the relatively large number of vacancies as well as early retirement. In this context, from a purely competitive point of view, an intercalated degree is less relevant. This is indeed true of some medical specialties, and thus doing an intercalated degree to give you an edge in the application process is simply not warranted. However, those going into general practice would still benefit from the other experiences and skills an intercalated degree provides.

An extra year

It take five years to complete the standard medical degree course, and hence studying for an extra year requires students to pay careful consideration to motivational, career and financial factors in order to make the right decision. The intercalated degree also comes hot on the heels of years 1 and 2, and thus you may be eager to get into clinics and see more patients.

Financial issues

With the introduction of means-tested tuition fees, student loans (rather than grants) and the reduction of funding from sponsors such as the Medical Research Council, one may conclude that there is little short-term financial incentive to gaining the extra degree. In a questionnaire study, 30 per cent of students stated that they would not do an intercalated degree for financial reasons, especially with the average final year medical student debt being £14 903 in 2002–3. Furthermore, you are another year away from qualifying to receive a proper salary, so you actually lose a year of earnings as well as paying an extra year's travel, living and textbook costs.

There are some mechanisms to offset some of these costs. If you do an intercalated degree your tuition fees will be paid in year 4 of the medical course. In addition, you will receive an NHS bursary of about £3000 or £5000, depending on whether you live with your parents or not (both the tuition fees and the bursary are normally only paid in year 5 – to prevent you from being penalized for doing a long course, compared to a 3-year BSc). You may be awarded funding to help with the costs of doing your intercalated degree. The PPP Foundation provides such funding to a small number of students – enquire at your medical school, as applications have to go through them and they recommend the students for the award. This can help to offset the aforementioned costs, but is only available for a few.

OTHER DISADVANTAGES

Other possible disadvantages include:

- Having to return to medicine upon completion of the intercalated degree, and the subsequent readjustment.
- Motivational difficulties.
- Being split from your friends if you don't do an intercalated degree (and they do).
- Some courses have very tough in-course components.
- Being in a laboratory on your own for many hours can be isolating.
- You may not be interested in doing research.
- The options available for intercalated degrees may not interest you, and some, such as tropical medicine, may not be available at your university.
- The knowledge acquired during an intercalated degree may be esoteric and not relevant to the medical degree or clinical practice.
- If you do an intercalated degree in history of medicine or another art, you may find the transition from medicine to art difficult.
- Watching some of your friends go 'one year ahead' by not doing an intercalated degree.

GREY AREAS

Subsequent performance in the rest of the medical degree

The content of intercalated degrees is often highly specialized and its long-term generic value is often questioned. Of course, doing an intercalated degree in anatomy is likely to be more useful for the rest of the medical course than one in the history of medicine. In terms of academic prowess, Tait and

Marshall (1995) found no consistent short-term correlation between doing an intercalated degree and subsequent marks in the clinical years. However, their study suffered from a small sample size (14 students), and adjustments for age and sex were not made.

Wyllie and Currie (1986) found that those who did an intercalated degree in pathology at Edinburgh did better in the remainder of the undergraduate curriculum than did their counterparts of equal academic ability who did not do an intercalated degree. However, this study was done when medical curricula and examinations included considerably more pathology. Furthermore, Mason and Scully (1987) found that 78 per cent of students who undertook intercalated degrees found them to be useful for the rest of the undergraduate course, although usefulness may not necessarily equate with higher marks in real terms.

A more recent study by Mohammad and Agha (2004) analysing the final year written paper results of 262 medical students at GKT showed that having previously done an intercalated degree was associated with a statistically significant higher exam mark, although this was found to be on average only 2.8 per cent greater. However, potential baseline differences in the two groups were not adjusted for (i.e. it may be that those who opt to do an intercalated degree in the first place are more intelligent/hard-working).

ALTERNATIVES TO DOING AN INTERCALATED DEGREE

Defer your decision until after clinical medicine begins

If you are still unsure about whether to do an intercalated degree, it might be worth considering continuing into clinical medicine and then intercalating between the third and fourth or fourth and fifth years of study. The advantages are that you will have more time to evaluate the different options for an intercalated degree, more time to gauge your own interests, and the chance of making your research more clinically based. Your BSc can have a different angle, taking into account the clinical experiences you acquired in the preceding year(s). The drawback is splitting up your clinical years and losing contact with patients at a time when your clinical skills are developing. You may also find it more difficult to motivate yourself.

MBPhD

Several medical schools offer the opportunity to do an integrated MBPhD programme. This allows medical students to obtain a basic medical degree and a PhD in about seven or eight years. If you are sure about a career in academic medicine then this is an option worth considering, as it will take less time than doing the degrees separately, and the integrated nature of the degree minimizes the potential loss of clinical skills. Fast-track intercalated or integrated doctorates were found to be effective in developing research orientation and academic leadership in the USA and Canada. However, this option is only available for a few, and is often very competitive.

Master's degree post qualification

A part-time master's degree done immediately after qualification over a two-year period during your PRHO and SHO posts is another option (especially as you will have more spare time when new European legislation enforces a 48-hour maximum working week in 2009 – currently it's 56 hours). This will allow you to save a year by not doing the intercalated degree, and it will confer more 'points' in future applications for SHO or registrar jobs. You are also likely to choose a degree subject that is related more to your eventual specialty, and is likely to be more clinically relevant than an intercalated degree done after 2 years of medical school. At this stage of your career the networking potential and opportunities to launch parallel or portfolio careers are much greater, and the master's degree can be considered a stepping stone to these.

From the financial viewpoint the degree itself is likely to cost you more; however, you will be in a better position to deal with the costs as you will be working full-time, earning £35 000 or so gross (using day release, evening study or distance learning to complete the degree). You will also save by not having to pay for an extra year's living, travel and books costs as a student.

By not doing an intercalated degree and keeping this option open, you have the advantage of seeing whether an additional degree will help you get that job. You may get a job without ever needing to do a BSc or an MSc – after all, in career terms, choosing to do an intercalated degree is a calculation of its potential benefit in giving you a competitive edge in the application process. You may decide to go into a less competitive career (e.g. general practice) where a BSc is not relevant for getting a job, or you may have other achievements which give you a good chance of getting a competitive job without needing to spend a year getting an intercalated degree. These calculations are best made nearer the time, as you may not know what your professional interests will be four or five years from now. If you find you come up against a 'glass ceiling' because, you feel, you don't have a BSc you can always do a master's degree at that time and be in the same year group as those who originally did an intercalated degree (or do it part time and stay one year ahead of their original peers). The downside is that doing a part-time master's degree requires self-discipline, good motivation, and the ability to work and study efficiently.

SOURCES OF FURTHER INFORMATION

Informal discussions with senior students and staff are vital for your information-gathering process. You need to ask specific questions, though, relating more to the programme you are interested in. What was it like, what skills and knowledge do students acquire, etc? Different people will provide different insights and viewpoints on what it is like to do that particular intercalated degree. Most of the relevant material available on the StudentBMJ, BMJ Careers and BMJ Classified websites has been summarized or referred to in this chapter, but it may be worth checking these sites to see if any recent material has been added. Many intercalated degree programmes may have their own website where more detailed information is available. Be wary of generalizations made by careers advisers and senior doctors at large conferences or meetings – their analysis of intercalated degrees is often rather black or white. This is a complex decision and you should weight their assessments proportionately in your overall information-gathering process.

CONCLUSION

The decision as to whether to do an intercalated degree is an individual one: there is no right or wrong answer. There are, however, two ways to do an intercalated degree – 'going with the flow' and simply getting a BSc in itself, or grabbing the bull by the horns and maximizing the personal and professional return on your investment of time, money and hard work. Endless arguments in numerous publications/fora will rage on because the authors/presenters are asking the wrong question: should *we* be doing intercalated degrees? Rather, you should ask, should *I* do an intercalated degree? You must weigh up all the potential benefits and drawbacks, consider the other available options, look at your individual situation and potential future career, and decide whether it's right for you.

SOURCES OF FUNDING

If you are accepted on an intercalated BSc programme, your arrangements for paying tuition fees will continue as normal – you will still have living costs and educational costs (book purchases, equipment, etc.).

Eligibility for an NHS bursary

Doing an intercalated BSc will entitle you to an NHS bursary from year 4 onwards, instead of from year 5. Currently, this amounts to between £3000 and £5000, depending on whether you live with your parents or not.

The hardship fund and loan

The hardship fund is money given to universities to help students in need. It is a grant and is not repayable. The hardship loan is provided on top of your student loan and is repayable just like the loan. You can apply for either of these through your college (applications forms are present at the Registry and the Student Welfare Office).

External awards

Such awards are usually administered by research or clinical associations/societies as well as by charities. A list of some of the external awards available is given in Appendix I.

REFERENCES AND FURTHER READING

Chambler AF, Chapman-Sheath PJ, Pearse MF. A model curriculum vitae: what are the trainers looking for? *Hospital Medicine* 1998; **59**: 324–6.

Eaton YT. The bachelor of medical science research degree as a start for clinician-scientists. *Medical Education* 1985; **19**: 445–51.

Evered JA, Griggs P, Wakeford R. The correlates of research success. *British Medical Journal* 1987; **295**: 241–6.

Galasko CS, Smith K. Ratio of basic surgical trainees to type 1 specialist registrar programmes 1999/2000/2001/2002. *Annals of the Royal College of Surgeons of England* 1999; **81** (3 Suppl): 124–8.

Greenhalgh T, Wong G. Doing an intercalated BSc can make you a better doctor. *Medical Education* 2003; **37**(9): 760–1.

London Deanery. NHS London. http://www.londondeanery.ac.uk/

McManus IC, Richards P, Winder BC. Intercalated degrees, learning styles, and career preferences: prospective longitudinal study of UK medical students. *British Medical Journal* 1999; **319**: 542-6.

Mason DK, Scully C. The intercalated honours BSc for dental students: a retrospective study. *British Dental Journal* 1987; **62**: 366-s8.

Mohammad S, Agha R. Are intercalated degrees associated with higher marks in clinical exams? Association of Medical Education, Liverpool, UK, 2 September 2004 (oral and poster).

Tait N, Marshall T. Is an intercalated BSc degree associated with higher marks in examinations during the clinical years? *Medical Education* 1995; **29**: 216-19.

Wyllie AH, Curry A. The Edinburgh intercalated honours BSc in pathology: evaluation of selection methods, undergraduate performance and postgraduate career. *British Medical Journal* 1986; **292**: 1646-8.

6

HOW TO ORGANIZE A SUCCESSFUL ELECTIVE

Riaz Agha

Electives have formed part of the medical course for 30 years now, and their importance is recognized in the GMC (2003) report *Tomorrow's Doctors*. They are a fantastic opportunity to broaden your experience and work in a different environment. They also represent an opportunity for you to distinguish yourself from fellow students and increase your chances of getting a competitive job.

There are two main of choices to make with regard to electives: what to do and where to go. Some students decide where they want to go first, and then decide on what they want to do (the specific specialty, and whether they want to gain mainly clinical or research experience). Others decide what to do first and then where they want to go. You should make this decision based on what is most important to you, what experiences you want, and what you think will most help you get ahead.

DO YOUR RESEARCH

The golden rule is to start researching early, at least a year before the expected date of your departure. Ideally you will have some idea of the specialty you want to do by the time you come to planning your elective. If, for example, you knew you wanted to do dermatology for your career, then ask several dermatologists at all grades what they think would be a good elective (where to go and what to do). You should also consult senior students who have already completed an elective, as well as reading their formal reports submitted to the medical school, which should be available in your library or online. Ask your personal tutor for advice, and generally get as many opinions as possible.

You can also consult a variety of websites for further information on specific electives, such as:

- The electives network http://www.the-mdu.com/studentm/ elective/student_network.
- Medical Electives http://www.medical-electives.com.
- Student BMJ http://www.studentbmj.com/international/ world.html.

Then, having written down these ideas and brainstormed yourself, have a good think about the options available and make a provisional decision.

WHAT TO DO?

There are essentially three main types of elective: clinical, research and specialist. Of course, the opportunities within these groups will be affected by the specialty you want to do and where you want to go. However, it is not necessary to narrow your choice down to a specific specialty: in many developing countries there is no significant degree of subspecialization, and you can get a broader experience in general medicine/surgery.

Clinical

These electives are concerned more with clinical experience, shadowing or embedding yourself in a clinical team and observing or getting involved with patient care. The degree to which you can get practically involved is highly variable, but generally tends to be greater in developing countries. You may use a clinical elective to give yourself experience of a particular specialty you are considering as a career choice. A clinical elective also allows you to make connections with consultants who may be able to offer advice if you decide to go and work or do research in that country in the future.

A clinical elective can also be used to help you contrast case loads and healthcare systems in different countries with those of the UK; you can also get a different perspective on the same specialty. For example, in the USA your experience may be more technological and investigation based, whereas in a developing country it may be more dependent on good clinical skills. During your elective you may have the opportunity to perform some clinical research, such as auditing the unit's figures, or even a questionnaire-based study involving patients. However, opportunities for laboratory research while undertaking clinical duties are rare.

Research

A research elective may be one of the few times in your life where you can dedicate yourself to producing a high-quality body of research without doing a higher degree. You will also have the opportunity to learn about research, study design, methods and practical techniques. It may also be possible to get your name on some of the research unit's papers, as well as present the research at international conferences: this would be a tremendous boost to your career and would raise your profile.

Doing a research elective also makes you eligible for a greater range of elective funding (see Appendix I). A string of research funding awards can look very good on your CV and provide a talking point in future job interviews. You may also pick up essential skills such as statistical and critical analysis, and important future research connections. In some specialties research experience looks very good on a CV: people will feel they are hiring the complete package, as very few applicants have significant research experience (validated by published papers, presentations and funding awards) and clinical experience (which you will get anyway as part of your regular medical training). Despite all the benefits, many people simply aren't interested in research and would not enjoy it; furthermore, some laboratories can be isolating.

It is advisable to go and visit the laboratory you are considering for your elective and meet your potential supervisor and colleagues, see the facilities and the nature of the research you will be doing: does it excite you? If possible, you should attempt to come away with the research proposal for the project you will be doing (this will outline the aims, rationale, hypothesis and experimental protocol for the project). Possession of this document will dramatically increase your chances of obtaining funding for your elective, as awarding committees will be able to see the cutting-edge research you will be doing and that you have it well planned – it's formal, and they know they will be getting their money's worth by funding you.

Most supervisors would not give this away by email, as it's a significant risk for them to give away research secrets and ideas to someone who may not even turn up: their research may involve unfiled patents, and so their intellectual property must be protected. By physically going there in your holidays you can demonstrate your enthusiasm and make a request (they are more likely to take you seriously if you do it that way). If for some reason you can't go well before your elective, try and get as much detail about the project via email or phone to build your own proposal.

Specialist

Specialist electives have become increasingly popular over the years as more diverse institutions take on elective students. Examples include working at NASA, sports medicine in Australia, wilderness medicine in Africa, scuba diving in the tropics, travel medicine and working with prison service doctors, to name but a few. These electives are aimed at giving you a completely different experience from standard 'career medicine'. They arouse great interest in those reading hundreds of CVs and will get you noticed. You will also be more likely to have the opportunity to write up such an elective for the popular medical media.

WHERE TO GO?

This is ultimately your choice, and there is no 'best' place to go. However, your decision on what to do will have an impact on where to do it. For example, if you wanted to do an elective in cardiology research, you might decide that the best centre for this is in the USA, perhaps the Mayo Clinic. On the other hand, you may have a burning desire to go somewhere completely different, such as rural China (just don't expect to find a cutting-edge centre there).

A fundamental choice is whether you want to go to the developed or the developing world (this is a very arbitrary distinction, and there is a large degree of variation). In a clinical elective you won't be able to do as much practical work in the developed world as in the developing. However, you may find that you become very frustrated or even panicked by the lack of equipment, drugs and teaching time in the developing world. At the same time, many students report how they find such situations exciting and the best part of their elective: they get to learn how much can be achieved with an enthusiastic team and basic nursing and medical care (Ismail, 2003).

Recently, Dr Matt Carty, Senior Vice-President and Overseas Officer at the Royal College of Obstetricians and Gynaecologists (RCOG), stated: 'I cannot stress how important it is to gain medical experience in an under-resourced country ... health systems are so different – there is bad obstetrics practice, overpopulation (Vanuatu has one doctor for 32 000 patients) and a wide range of diseases, and such a diverse range of people and cultures ... these placements are life-changing experiences.' Carty was referring to two schemes set up by the RCOG for doctors to obtain experience in developing countries (cited in Hall, 2004). This shows how seriously such work is viewed by one Royal College. As a medical student you will have greater autonomy, more decision-making, and will need to use your initiative more.

The elective will also help to place medicine in a broader sociopolitical context, and you will realize just how much health policy and budgets really matter. The unique experiences you would gain on elective would probably provide discussion points at future interviews: you must be able to state what your objectives were and what you learned, as well as to believe in them and say it passionately.

For a research elective, you are far more likely to find eminent scientists and world-renowned laboratories in the developed world (where you will also have a greater chance of publication, and so on). On the downside, they are unlikely to be involved in researching diseases that don't affect their own population in significant numbers. These are generalizations, but they are worth bearing in mind before conducting more specific research via books, the Internet, elective reports, and asking staff and older students.

When making your decisions, ask yourself the following questions:

- What specialty are you interested in?
- Do you want a clinical, research or specialist elective?
- Do you want to go to the developed or the developing world?
- How do you think you would cope there?
- What do you want to achieve? What are your specific objectives?

Of course, when you have two to three months or so for your elective, you can divide up your time and combine different kinds of electives and locations. However, this must be thought through, as you may not get a full experience at either location and may not fulfil your objectives. For a research elective, you need to maximize the amount of time you spend conducting research, otherwise your name may not be on the paper published by the unit. It is easier to do this for a clinical elective, comparing the developing and developed worlds, contrasting the two healthcare systems for the same specialty. Consult broadly and see what's possible and what you would enjoy doing. Whatever you do, make sure you keep a good log of your activities and take plenty of good photos for your report.

HOW TO APPLY FOR GRANT FUNDING

Funding an elective can be expensive. However, there are a large number of awards out there, many of which go unclaimed or receive little competition each year (see Appendix I for a list). However, before embarking on your funding applications, you should follow the process outlined below.

Basic questions to ask
- What is the nature of your research?
- Who would fund it?
- Who funds other researchers in this area?

The next step
- Do your grant research well ahead of time.
- Draw up a list of potential sponsors, their web addresses and their deadlines.
- Go to each site and ensure you meet the eligibility criteria.
- Download the application form and additional materials.

Build your proposal
Prepare the following standard documents:

- Covering letter
- Statement of intent

- Research proposal
- Budget.

If you need to have referees to support your application, approach them and obtain their consent – make sure they are willing to support your application.

You need to tailor each individual application to the aims and objectives of the individual sponsor/grant provider. Make sure your application fits within the overall research focus or strategy of the organization.

When applying to multiple sponsors, be careful that there are no rules/regulations whereby you can't be awarded multiple times for doing the same thing.

Ask others to read your proposal and make sure your research supervisor approves the documentation you send, and get their advice on how you can improve it (they may have concerns about intellectual property rights, as sending a proposal reveals their ideas, so always check first).

Apply

- Apply early.
- Send your applications by recorded or special delivery.

After sending in your application

Seek confirmation of receipt from the sponsor, and ensure that you keep their email on file.

HOW TO RESEARCH POTENTIAL SPONSORS

Search everywhere – electronic and human

Electronic searching

- Do an advanced search in Google for your area of research, e.g. 'wound healing' and 'funding' or 'sponsorship' or 'grant' or 'award'.
- Go to grant funding portals such as http://www.**grants.gov**.

Human searching

Consult broadly – ask colleagues and supervisors.

Remember

It is better to apply to more sponsors than to overly narrow down your search. For example, the following types of sponsor may be interested in providing grants to a wound healing research project that focuses on angiogenesis:

- Wound management associations
- Cancer research organizations
- The Wellcome Trust/Howard Hughes
- Microcirculation societies
- NASA
- Defence organizations
- American and British Associations of Plastic Surgery
- American and British Associations of Dermatology
- Diabetes UK/American Diabetes Association
- British Geriatrics Society
- European Society of Vascular Surgery
- Charities.

HOW TO BUILD YOUR STANDARD DOCUMENTS

Covering letter (one page)

Introduce yourself, your institution, the laboratory/unit and the research you are doing.

Statement of intent (1–2 pages)

When applying for an individual grant, in this section it is important to state:

- What you think you will gain from the research.
- How this will affect your personal development.
- What practical skills and knowledge you will learn.
- How you will benefit from interactions with the other members of the research team.

For a government grant a specific statement of intent as laid out above is not usually required.

Research proposal (2–5 pages)

This document should be broken down into the following sections:

- Details of the researchers and the institution.
- An abstract.
- Hypothesis and specific aims (state how long it will take to achieve your targets).
- Background, significance and rationale (including epidemiology and economic data, as well as an understanding of current approaches to the problem, avoid circular reasoning where the lack of your proposed solution is the problem).
- Preliminary studies and results.
- Research design and methods (in the context of your specific aims).
- Materials and method.
- Publications, presentation and awards of the research team (a demonstration of credibility).
- References.
- Appendix.

Budget

For a government grant include all costs for equipment and supplies projected over the course of the experimental period. For an individual grant make sure you include all travel, living and accommodation costs.

TIPS ON HOW TO HAVE A SMOOTH JOURNEY

Here are some of the things you should do before you go:

- Apply for your visa early. If you are going to the USA – you don't need one, just sign a visa waiver form and a customs declaration on the plane and that's it (only certain countries in addition to the UK are eligible: check on the US embassy site to be sure).

- Buy a digital camera and a 512 Mb or 1 GB memory card – you will save on film and development costs in the long term, plus there is no risk of your photos being ruined during development. Furthermore, if you take a laptop, you can upload the images directly, edit them and then send them straight away to your family.

- Scan important documents and then save them to a CD and email them to yourself. If anything goes wrong you can retrieve them easily.

- Make sure you have enough money in your bank account and enough credit on your credit cards to ensure that you get through the elective without financial problems.

- Always expect to come back heavier, so make sure you have enough spare room in your suitcases and make sure your luggage does not go overweight for the journey back (check with your airline about weight limits for baggage and hand luggage).

- Stick some thick silver tape or even a ribbon to your luggage to prevent anyone else picking up your bags on the baggage carousel.

- Have an aspirin on the day of the flight (if you are concerned about 'economy class syndrome').

- Go vegetarian (inform your travel agent in advance): you will get your meal well before anyone else and will maximize your time to do other things.

- Search around for a good exchange rate on foreign currency.

- Make sure you have enabled Internet banking on your current account so you can check up on your balance and pay bills (most of which you should place on direct debit) while you are abroad.

- Make sure all of your ongoing bills (mobile, Internet access, contact lenses, etc.) are paid by direct debit.

- If you are going to a country with a high HIV rate, make sure you pack a HIV post-exposure prophylaxis (PEP) starter pack.

- You cannot buy anything online or over the phone in the USA using a UK credit card. It is therefore advisable to open a bank account and get a debit card while you are on elective. There may be similar situations in other countries.
- The best way to get cash abroad is via cash machines bearing the 'Maestro' or 'Cirrus' signs. If your debit card bears these symbols, you will be charged less than the cost of changing money at a bank or doing a bank transfer (and you will tend to get a more favourable exchange rate).

REFERENCES AND FURTHER READING

National Office for Statistics. Census 2001. http://www.statistics. gov.uk/census2001/default.asp – this link will help you to draw comparisons between your potential destination and the UK in terms of demographics – it will help to reference this when write your elective report as well.

Centre for Disease Control and Prevention. Department of Health and Human Services. http://www.cdc.gov/ – get information on disease prevalence in the UK.

Dick E. Observership – what is it and how can I do one? *BMJ Careers* 2003; **327**: s73–4.

Electives – raising the cash. http://www.traumaroom.com/uk/9/ page12.html

Foreign and Commonwealth Office. http://www.fco.gov.uk – to find out about the latest travel warnings (your medical school may not let you go to areas of conflict).

General Medical Council. *Tomorrow's Doctors*. London: General Medical Council, 2003.

Hall S. Developing world to develop your career. *Hospital Doctor* 2004; 10 June: 30.

Health Statistics Quarterly. http://www.hic.gov.au/statistics/dyn_ std/forms/monqtr4.shtml

International Health Exchange. http://www.ihe.org.uk – provides contacts to organizations which work in developing countries.

Ismail Y. The way I see it: Working in a developing country is a positive experience. *BMJ Careers* 2003; **327**: s14.

Lonely Planet. http://www.medical-electives.com – Travel Guides.

Map Quest. http://www.medical-electives.com – Travel Guides.

Masta: Mind your health abroad. http://www.masta.org/ – practical health advice.

Medics Travel. http://www.medicstravel.com – consult this for a list of hospital contacts, non-governmental organizations and charities.

StudentBMJ. http://www.studentbmj.com/international/ world.html – read elective reports on places that interest you.

Voluntary Services Overseas. http://www.vso.org.uk – an international development charity that works through volunteers.

World Health Organization. http://www.who.int/en/ – use this to research the prevalence of different diseases in a country.

GETTING AHEAD OF THE COMPETITION

7

HOW TO GET SHORTLISTED FOR COMPETITIVE JOBS

Riaz Agha

Progressing up the medical career ladder is a tough business. Many candidates find themselves waiting years for specialty training posts, before their applications are considered strong enough for them to be invited to interview, let alone given a job. The candidates who are most likely to be successful in getting such jobs in a highly competitive environment are those that knew what they had to do well ahead of time (and did it!). This chapter will tell what you need to know to give yourself the best chance of getting a competitive post. Furthermore, you should attempt to achieve most of these while you are at medical school.

WHAT ARE THEY LOOKING FOR?

In short, many things, the reason being that you have to distinguish yourself. Getting your medical degree, getting an intercalated degree and good references won't distinguish you significantly from the crowd (see Chapter 5). So, what exactly can you do to increase your chances?

Published scientific papers

The phrase *'publish or perish'* was coined because of the intense pressure felt by individuals to get scientific papers published or 'perish' in career terms. Ideally, your research (from an intercalated BSc, an SSM, or another project of your own initiative) should be published in journals that are indexed by databases such as Medline and PubMed (these databases contain over 3000 journals).

Don't panic if your research gets an absolute rejection by such journals (i.e. without the opportunity for a revision): if you can't improve your paper any further, try getting it published in a non-indexed journal – they don't look as impressive, but they still count. You can also try submitting your research as a short communication or a letter. Publishing letters and case reports is an easier way of building your confidence and will confer credit to you in any case. Be prepared for rejection: I was rejected many times before I got my first paper published, and be assured that this is the norm. Once my first paper was published, I realized that while I was being rejected I was actually progressing along a learning curve for the principle 'selecting the right manuscript for the right journal'. If you start submitting research during your earlier years of medical school, you get through this learning curve while you are still there. Always pay attention to the comments you get back from editors, respect them and learn from them (see Chapter 8).

Audit projects

This is where you compare observed clinical practice and results (which you record objectively) with the reference best-practice guidelines developed for that disease (such guidelines may be available from the National Institute of Clinical Excellence (NICE) or a specialty's professional association). For example, you may look at how many doctors wash their hands between seeing patients on a particular ward, and compare with the national guidelines that every doctor should wash their hands between seeing every patient. Audits help to improve adherence to a 'best' reference standard of practice. At the end of the audit you make recommendations on what can be done to improve adherence to the standard. Following implementation of these recommendations you can come back and redo the audit to see whether implementation of the changes you recommended made any difference to the outcomes. This is called 'closing the audit loop', and people want to see that you closed the audit loop when you write audit projects on your CV.

Presentations

Presentations of research work at local, regional, national and international conferences can be a good boost to a CV and show that you take part in the wider scientific and clinical community; they also help to raise your profile and give you a more respectable name. When choosing which conference to submit your work to for presentation, either as a poster or orally (oral presentations are worth more), look to see which ones will publish an abstract of your work in a supplementary issue of a journal. An abstract goes on your publication record and helps to add further clout to your CV (you can still do the presentation and publish the full paper in another journal if you wish, so consider this a bonus).

Medical school prizes, distinctions and scholarships

There are large numbers of these available at your medical school, so you should do your best to seek them out and submit for them. Check all the medical noticeboards and with your registry. Search the web for prizes that are external to your institution. For example, you could do an advanced search on www.teoma.com for 'prize' or 'scholarship' and 'your medical school name'. Also, try to get as many prizes and awards as possible for your intercalated BSc (if you choose to do one) and your elective (see Appendix I).

Management experience

At medical school this is manifest as being President of a Surgical Society, or being involved with your Students' Union (as a house officer, it's called being Mess President). Being effective in positions of responsibility demonstrates your leadership qualities to potential employers. Such positions require you to know how to manage your time, be able to communicate effectively, and to get results through the responsible and efficient delegation of tasks (see Chapter 2, 'Time management').

Teaching experience

Throughout your training as a clinician you will also be teaching those more junior than you. Thus teaching skills and experience are viewed favourably. There are often groups of medical students who teach cardiopulmonary resuscitation (CPR) or suturing skills to other students: join them and learn how to teach – it's not easy, and you need to appreciate the principles involved. In fact, trying to teach and explain complex things in a way other people can understand will develop your communication skills and help to add logic and clarity to your thought processes. Again, this comes back to wanting and needing to develop yourself as an individual.

Elective experience

A unique and worthwhile elective from which you gain useful amounts of knowledge, skills and attitudes will demonstrate your ability to cope with diversity and with a different healthcare environment (see Chapter 6).

Non-medical experience and qualifications

These can demonstrate that you are a well-rounded individual with a broad view of life, as well as an appreciation of what learning new concepts and types of knowledge can do for your efficiency. Qualifications in the realm of information technology, such as the European Computer Driving Licence (ECDL; http://www.ecdl.com) are particularly useful (see Chapter 3). You should also demonstrate your personality and individuality by maintaining involvement with extracurricular activities that interest you (everyone wants to work with an interesting and charismatic person).

Later on, as a house officer, you will be required to know more about clinical governance, as well as have a greater awareness of evidence-based practice and broader issues in the NHS. As a medical student you can start reading about these issues to build up your knowledge, as you are likely to be questioned on such areas eventually.

Ultimately, doing your best to get shortlisted using the advice above will actually end up making you a better doctor. This is exactly why this forms the criteria for shortlisting – those who have been successful in these areas make well-rounded and efficient clinicians who are able to deal with a broad array of challenges, situations and professional commitments (as most consultants do on a daily basis, for example).

FURTHER READING

London Deanery. http://www.londondeanery.ac.uk/ – this site contains person specification criteria and provides more information on what you should do to increase your chances of getting a job once you qualify.

8

HOW TO WRITE AND PUBLISH A SCIENTIFIC PAPER

Riaz Agha

Writing and publishing scientific papers is one of the most important activities for your career progression. When you are applying for basic specialist training posts, the number of papers on your CV will be a key way of distinguishing you from candidates. Those who are 'well published' have conducted research or reviewed an area of the literature to a high standard. In fact, the phrase 'publish or perish' has increasingly been used to describe the urgency and value of publishing papers for one's career.

Fortunately, so many medical journals now exist that your chances of publishing good work are relatively high. Always ask yourself what message you have and which journal would be most appropriate? Do you want to write it for a generalist audience or a specialist audience? Whichever you decide, the paper you write must be well written and constructed in the conventional manner. You must always pay close attention to the 'Instructions to authors' for the particular journal you are submitting to. Some journals may reject your paper simply for not following their procedures; at the very least it will count against you in the assessment.

After reading your research paper, an individual should be able to:

- Assess the observations you have made.
- Have sufficient details to be able to repeat the experiment (if they wish).
- Determine whether the conclusions you have made are objectively justified by your results.

Following a short abstract, most manuscripts and journals follow this structure:

- **Introduction** – what are you investigating and why? This should ideally be encapsulated in a series of questions you hope to answer by conducting your research.
- **Methods** – how you chose to investigate the questions you have posed.
- **Results** – what did you find?
- **Discussion** – What do your findings mean?

It is advisable to keep a folder of good scientific papers published in well-renowned international journals to serve as examples on structure and layout. Now let's look at each of these sections in more detail.

Introduction

The main purpose of the introduction is to tell the reader concisely why you chose to undertake the study: you should provide the thought process that led you to ask the key question(s) in the study, and why these are significant (it is often useful to cite some epidemiological facts here). You need to review the relevant literature on the subject and show that past studies (or lack of them) have led you to ask these question(s). You will need to cite the references that support your analysis – usually three citations from different groups are enough to convince reviewers that a fact is 'well recognized' (especially if they are from different countries).

You should also clarify what your work could add to the existing body of knowledge.

You should also be aware of the suggested structures for certain kinds of study: these allow for greater standardization and prevent important information being omitted. Guidelines have now been created for:

- Randomized controlled trials (Moher *et al.*, 2001)
- Systematic reviews (Moher *et al.*, 1999)
- Economic evaluations (Drummond and Jefferson, 1996)
- Diagnostic method reports (Bossuyt *et al.*, 2003).

Many journals now require you to stick to these guidelines and will send back papers that don't conform. At the end of your introduction, you should have a sentence which leads the reader into the study design proper, e.g. 'We therefore decided to undertake a randomized controlled trial with 20 years' follow-up to see if high-heeled shoes increased the risk of developing arthritis'.

Methods

A poor Methods section is the most common reason for the absolute rejection of a paper. The purpose of this section is to describe your experimental design and, if appropriate, to provide the rationale for using it. You should provide enough information for someone else to repeat your experiment: this will help to guide you on how much detail you should provide. If you have used standard methods, then reference them. If you have used methods that are not standard but have been used by another group, then read their Methods section and see how they described the technique.

This section will also cover the statistical methods you used to analyse your results (state which software package and version you used). It is best to consult a statistician before you embark on your study. Find out what they think about your study and its design: they will provide advice on how you can maximize the chances of getting results which are valid and which could be analysed professionally. It is difficult for them to give such advice after a poorly designed study has already been carried out. It is critically important not to introduce too many unknowns into your methods: look at one thing at a time, so you can isolate association, cause and effect sensibly.

Results

The aim of the Results section is to describe what you found, especially the major findings of the study. The data should be presented in the most appropriate and useful way for the reader. You should only present relevant data (which refers to the question posed in the introduction). Think about how you can best present it, in tables and graphs (as if telling a story). Remember, most people will skip straight to the tables and graphs without reading all the text (don't forget to mention the units in table columns). It might also be useful to state the important negatives – what you didn't find – just to help clarify your results. The Results section does not usually require referencing or any interpretation of data.

For a study involving participants, you would usually begin with a description of your sample (age, sex, and so on) to show how representative it is. You should aim to address one topic per paragraph, from most important to least important. Try to emphasize the most important results by making short, sharp and definitive statement about them (do not use table or figure legends for these). Try to avoid ambiguous statements, such as 'A' decreased compared with 'B', as this does not tell you whether 'B' changed or stayed the same. It is better to say 'A' decreased more than 'B', or even more precise would be 'A decreased whereas 'B' remained unchanged (use the past tense, as the event has already happened).

Don't confuse significance with statistical significance. In fact, it's better not to use the word 'significance' in the Results section (this is an individual's qualitative judgement), unless you are saying statistical significance (where you would also give a p-value). To describe a perceived 'big' change, use the word 'markedly'. Furthermore, just because a hormone level's rise is statistically significant, does not mean it will be biologically significant (i.e. it will not cause a measurable clinical effect).

Discussion

The aims of this section are as follows:

- Summarize your major findings.
- Interpret your findings and put them in the context of the existing literature.
- What is their significance in scientific and clinical terms?
- Discuss any doubts, weaknesses and confounders.
- Discuss the limitations of your methods and your study.
- Suggest further work.
- Produce a tightly worded and precise conclusion.

The problem with the Discussion section is that it can often become very long-winded. In general, it should not be more than one-third of the total length of the paper. You might find it helpful just to write it out in its entirety and then cut it down afterwards.

Most discussions start with either the main finding from the study, a mini-review of the field, or what's different about the present study. My personal preference is to start with the main finding from the study, as the other techniques tend to lead to repetition of the Introduction. Most discussions finish with any of these three conclusions: 'gap filled', 'more research is needed' or 'uncertainty remains'. This will of course depend on the results and the conclusions you have drawn from them.

The most common errors include repeating parts of your Results section; confusing association with cause and effect, a failure to discuss studies that don't support your conclusions, stating conclusions that are not supported by your data, and a failure to identify the limitations of your methods.

OTHER ASPECTS

Other important aspects of the manuscript are the title and the abstract. In addition, following your discussion you should acknowledge those who helped the study reach completion (e.g. those who provided information, technical or statistical help, as well as patients who took part in trials – but be careful never to give their names). You should also never say 'I' in a paper: if you wish to refer to one of the authors it's better to say 'one of us'). The References section is also a common site for mistakes: unfortunately, there is a wide variety of reference styles, so always check the instructions to authors and have a look at the papers the journal has published previously. Don't just cite reviews that agree with you – cite some of the important original research studies that the review was based on. There is also no need to cite very large numbers of studies, as this shows insecurity. It's better to pick out the most important studies that most relate to the point you are making. What is the word limit for the type of article you want to submit (check the instructions to authors)?

You will usually have to submit a covering letter with your paper. This should ideally state that your work has not been published previously and not co-submitted elsewhere. You also need to state who funded the study, and whether there are any conflicts of interest. For multi-author papers you will also have to state the role played by each in the study. Once you have finished writing your paper, ask your supervisor and someone not connected with the project to review it for you prior to submission to a journal. It's amazing how many errors can be eliminated at this late stage.

REFERENCES

Bossuyt PM, Reitsma B, Bruns DE *et al.* Towards complete and accurate reporting of studies of diagnostic accuracy: the STARD initiative. *British Medical Journal* 2003; **326**: 41–4.

Drummond MF, Jefferson TO. Guidelines for authors and peer-reviewers of economic submissions to the BMJ. The BMJ Economic Evaluation Working Party. *British Medical Journal* 1996; **313**: 275–83.

Moher D, Cook DJ, Eastwood S *et al.* Improving the quality of reports of meta-analyses of randomised controlled trials: the QUOROM statement. Quality of Reporting Meta-analyses. *Lancet* 1999; **354**: 1896–900.

Moher D, Schulz KF, Altman DG. The CONSORT statement: revised recommendations for improving the quality of reports of parallel-group randomised trials. *Lancet* 2001; **357**: 1191–4.

9

HOW TO PUBLISH YOUR OWN BOOK

Mohammad Al-Ubaydli

One of the pleasures of my college library was coming across books such as *Queueing Systems: Vol.1: Theory.* It was comforting to know that a topic I had never given a second thought to still had experts to document it in several volumes. The beauty of modern publishing is that it allows authors in increasingly specialized fields to share their knowledge with the rest of the world. As readers, doctors and patients, we are all beneficiaries of these fruits of knowledge expansion.

However, the system is not yet perfect. Although almost anyone can be an expert on something, not everyone can have his or her book published. The costs of paper, printing, distribution and marketing mean that a minimum number of potential readers must be found before a publisher will invest money in a book. Perhaps this is a good thing – traditional publishers will tell you that the world is spared many an unreadable text because of such a barrier, and they are indeed correct. But I also think that too many good books take too long to reach readers because of traditional publishers. This chapter provides you with a gradual series of steps to overcome this barrier.

A fast and affordable way to start off is to create a website. If that goes well, the next step is to write a complete book. New technology makes it relatively cheap and easy to print a book.

Finally, you can start your own publishing business and bring your book to the world. This chapter will take you through the entire process, and I hope that you have as much fun as I did when I followed these steps and published my own book.

WORLD WIDE WHAT?

It is extremely difficult to do a search on the Internet and get no results at all. Whatever topic you can think of, it is likely that lots of people have already had lots of things to say about it. The miracle of the World Wide Web is that they can get to say these things so easily, and that you can read them so easily.

There are several steps to contributing to the web. First, you need to write something using web-authoring software. Next, you must make this writing available to others using a website. Finally, you must let the rest of the world know about your website. All these steps are easy and affordable.

Step 1 – the write software

If you have a word processor, for example Microsoft Word or Open Office (which is free from http://www.openoffice.org), then you are ready to go. Start writing as you would with any document. The trick is to save the document as a web page. Click on the 'File' menu, choose 'Save as web page. . .' and click on the 'Save' button. That's it: you have created your first web page.

Creating a web page is easy, but creating a good one takes a little more thought. This is because 'people rarely read Web pages word by word; instead, they scan the page, picking out individual words and sentences' (http://www.useit.com/alertbox/9710a.html). A good web author makes it easy for the reader to scan the text. Use short clear sentences, big clear headings, break up the text into separate pages, and connect them using hypertext links.

Hypertext link is the technical term for the line that you see under words on a web page. When you click on such words, your web browser takes you to another page. Using such links allows the reader to move quickly between different parts of your text, allowing them to navigate according to their interests. You can create links using Microsoft Word, but the program was not really designed for this.

There are many good examples of serious and popular web-authoring software out there, including NVU (which is available free from http://www.nvu.com) and Microsoft FrontPage (with an interface that is similar to Word). However, if you are just beginning, consider CuteSite Builder (www.globalscape.com/cutesitebuilder). This program makes it easy for anyone to create a good website. It takes you painlessly through all the steps, and instills good habits. At $115.00 (about £70), it's worth the investment just to get the excellent technical support. I used it for most of my websites, including my personal one, http://www.mo.md.

For advanced users, the gold standard is Macromedia DreamWeaver. Of course, it costs far more than CuteSite (about £250) and is only worth getting if you will spend a lot of time on an advanced website. It was the natural choice when I designed the *Medical Approaches* (http://www.medicalapproaches.org) and *Handhelds Computers for Doctors* (http://www.handheldsfordoctors.com) websites.

Step 2 – share the literature

Once you have created your web page, you need a place on the web to put it (a website) and a way to transfer it to there. Most Internet service providers (ISPs), such as Freeserve, AOL and Tiscali, already provide you with such a place free of charge. If your ISP does not do this, companies such as Tripod (http://www.tripod.com) and Bizland (http://www.bizland.com) also offer websites for free. You can pay them, or other companies such as Pair (http://www.pair.com), for more services. The companies can also supply you with your own custom web address – for example http://www.mo.md, rather than http://www.bizland.com/mo.

On the Internet, the protocol for transferring files is called file transfer protocol (FTP) and various FTP programs are available. You will need such a program to transfer your web page from your computer to your website. SmartFTP (http://www.smartftp.com) is one such program and is free for personal and educational use, and it does the job admirably. Even better, most specialized web authoring programs have FTP facilities; these include CuteSite Builder, which makes the whole transfer process delightfully simple.

Step 3 – build it, and they will come

Having a website is good, but knowing that people are making use of it is great. People will hear about a website in three ways: through friends' recommendations; through web searches; and through web links. You must work on all three ways to spread the word.

In the beginning, personal recommendations will be your commonest source of traffic. So, tell all your family, friends and colleagues about the website. Include your website address on your business card. A great way to subtly remind people is to include it at the bottom of every email you write. This latter technique is so powerful that it is credited with getting Hotmail its first 30 million customers in just 30 months, so use it.

Second, you must make sure that search engines are well aware of your website. These include Google (http://www.google.com), Yahoo! (http://www.yahoo.com) and MSN (http://www.msn.com), and each has a slightly different way of adding your website to its list. Search Engine Watch (http://www.searchenginewatch.com) provides an excellent guide to the steps involved.

However, just being on the list does not mean that you will be high on that list – to get there, you need the web equivalent of the peer review process. If other websites find your website useful, they make links to it. The more links going to your website, the more useful it is to the searcher, and the higher up the list you climb.

A quick way to get started is to join a web ring. This is a set of sites covering a single topic that agree to provide links to each other. For example, if your website is about cystic fibrosis, do a search on Google for 'cystic fibrosis web ring'. This brings up an excellent site (http://www.azcowboy88.tripod.com/welcome/ which is hosted on Tripod) that you can join. For a more time-consuming but longer-lasting way, get personal. Again, if your website is about cystic fibrosis, search for 'cystic fibrosis' top of the list. Visit those sites and try to find the email address of the person running them. Tell them about your site, and ask if they would include a link to it.

The web is built on such personal contact, so make sure that your own website also includes an email address. With time you will be getting emails from grateful readers, impressed colleagues and, of course, new website owners who see you as part of the web establishment. Congratulations – you are now a web publisher.

WRITING YOUR BOOK

A website is a great way to start sharing your knowledge and skills. As the text that you have begins to accumulate, however, it becomes more useful to your readers as a book. There is also a phenomenal sense of satisfaction to be derived from saying 'have you read my book', although best of all is being able to carry your own book around with you and being able to show it off with pride.

Books about writing books

In many newspapers today you will find small adverts for books that explain a get-rich-quick scheme. Each scheme will be different, but apparently the surest scheme is to write a book about getting rich. Similarly, many of the richest authors are those that write books explaining how to write books.

Nevertheless, many of these books are very useful. One that constantly dominates the bestseller list is *The Self-Publishing Manual* (Poynter, 2003). Already in its 13th edition, its author wrote his first book, the *Parachute Manual*, because he thoroughly enjoyed his new hobby of parachuting but could not find a good textbook on the topic. I found *The Self-Publishing Manual* to be extremely useful as it gave me a good overview of the full process, explained where to look for detailed information, and most of all, helped me believe that it was possible to do all this alone.

Tools to use

Write your book using a computer. No matter how tempting you find a typewriter, comfortable you feel with paper, or intimidated you are by computers, make sure you use a computer for this job. If you want to improve your typing skills, consider using a program such as Mavis Beacon Teaches Typing (http://www.mavisbeacon.com). Most computer shops sell copies of the software, and occasionally computer magazines give away free copies. Of course your typing will naturally improve with practice, and working as a medical secretary during your holidays can be invaluable here.

As you might expect, there is a wide range of software to choose from. This includes 'professional' software such as Quark Xpress or Adobe Indesign. However, if you are starting out you should use the word processing software that came with your computer, such as Microsoft Word. If you do not have any of this, get Open Office, an excellent and comprehensive software suite that is available free of charge.

Most word processors have excellent tools for dealing with large amounts of text such as a book. They will allow you to divide the book into sections, chapters and subsections; they will keep track of all your references, footnotes and endnotes; and they can deal with layout and diagrams. As long as your book does not have too many diagrams, word processors such as Open Office or Microsoft Word are all that you need.

Timing

Some authors claim that anyone can write a book within 14 days, even while holding a day job. Perhaps this is true, and perhaps finding out how to do this is a good reason to pay the money to attend courses that teach this. However, in my experience such a deadline is ambitious. Give yourself time, and ideally make it uninterrupted time, such as a holiday. In my case, it was a great way to make use of a short period of unemployment.

Having said that, it is still useful to have a deadline. Your brain will always come up with reasons why it shouldn't do a bit of writing today, and a deadline is often the only counter-argument.

Finally, there are several small tasks that involve other people, and which can thus greatly lengthen the time until your book is ready for publication. These include having colleagues proofread your book, getting an ISBN number (see below), and coordinating a printer. However, you can do many of these in parallel with your writing, so a little planning saves a great deal of time.

Proofreading

You can save money by making use of friends and colleagues to help with this. Many amateur heads are better than one, so give each proofreader a small section. To speed things up, send the sections out as soon as you finish them, even as you continue to write more sections. Give the proofreaders advance warning about the date when you expect to send out a section, and ask them to devote a block of time for the task. Finally, make use of the 'track changes' feature in your word processor. In Microsoft Word this is available in the 'Tools' menu, whereas in Open Office it is in the 'Edit' menu.

If you are lucky, you will be friends with an editor, and they will be an excellent resource.

ISBN

The international standard book number (ISBN) is a unique identifier for every book around the world and helps buyers, sellers and publishers communicate. Getting an ISBN for your book takes a little effort and a little money, but most of all it takes time for all your paperwork to be processed, so it is one of those jobs that you should do as soon as possible.

Start by visiting the ISBN Agency's excellent website (www.whitaker.co.uk/newpublishers.htm) and register through their Standard Service. The fee is £60.00 + VAT, and it gets you 10 ISBN numbers. You can then apply these to any 10 books that you publish. If you publish more, you can buy more numbers in blocks of 100 or more (depending on how ambitious you feel), but you cannot buy individual numbers.

This is extremely supportive pricing. Think of Hermann Hauser, the Austrian-born entrepreneur. He moved to the UK and founded a string of companies, including Acorn Computers in 1978. He said that he did so because it cost just £100 to register with Company House. At these prices, everyone should try their hand.

Cover design

Barnes and Noble is America's largest bookseller. According to industry legend, if you think a book shouldn't be judged by its cover, then you have not met the buyer from Barnes and Noble. This is a little unfair, but only because the company is not the only one that has this practice. Your book's cover is very important, and everyone from the bookstore manager to the final reader will base a large part of their buying decisions on how much they like it. So, get a good cover. If you have artistically talented friends, ask for their help. Look at other books for inspiration on good cover design, do web searches for ideas on images, and think seriously about getting a professional to design the cover.

PRINTING YOUR BOOK

A good printer is like a good plumber: their costs and results, as well as the reliability of the person you are dealing with, can vary considerably.

A good starting point is the London Book Fair, where many printers display their samples. Alternatively, searching on the web or asking colleagues at universities should get you some phone numbers or email addresses. No matter how you find them, printers will always send you free sample copies to show you the quality of their work. Take advantage of these and compare what is on offer.

For your first book, a short print run is probably the best way to go. The printing costs quite a bit more per copy, but you can print a more manageable load. Printers unable to provide short runs usually require that you print over a thousand copies, and the total bill can make your venture risky. What would you do if you were left with 950 unsold copies?

Talking to a printer requires practice, and it is possible to be taken advantage of if you appear naive to the business. So it is worthwhile getting a book that you like, and talking about it to a printer that you don't like. Ask them how to make an exact copy of the book, and note down what words they use to describe it. This is the language you will need to regurgitate as you talk to the next printer.

In addition, there are three subtle items that you should make sure your printer is able to do. First, they must accept electronic copies of the book. In other words, they must be able to work from an electronic file that you send them, rather than demanding that you print out the book and mail it. This is one of the key advantages of using a computer to write the book, and if your printer cannot continue the process then you should not trust their competence. Second, make sure that they can generate and print the ISBN and barcode on to the back of your book cover. No bookseller will agree to stock your book otherwise, and few readers will take it seriously. Finally, ask for the copies to be shrink-wrapped. It will cost a little extra, but it adds professionalism to your efforts and ensures that the book arrives in good condition to your readers.

SELLING YOUR BOOK

There is a great feeling that comes from seeing your name in print, and many authors consider this to be the well-deserved end of their toils. However, to borrow the words of Sir Winston Churchill: 'this is not the end. It is not even the beginning of the end. But it is, perhaps, the end of the beginning'. If you are serious about getting people to read the knowledge that you have worked so hard to accumulate and document, then there is a lot of work yet to be done.

Getting the word out

Printing costs money, but it is only a small part of a book's price. The main costs are for marketing and distribution. Marketing is not just about advertising, it is about the larger task of making sure the right person knows that your product is right for them. For example, if you make medication for cardiac patients, and most cardiac patients are elderly, good marketing means that your leaflets should be in large print.

The first step in getting the word out about your book is getting good reviews. This is tricky, but do not be shy about approaching the highest authority in your book's field. The worst they can do is say they are too busy, but most are surprisingly helpful. What you need is one good review from one good authority so that you can put it on the back of your cover. Be persistent.

When your book is available for sale, and you have acquired good reviews, it is time for a press release. This is a concise and detailed document that explains to a member of the press why their readers would be interested to know about your book, and how to contact you to get more information. A good place to learn more about writing press releases is the PRW website (http://www.press-release-writing.com).

Handling the sales

A few days after I sent out press releases about my book from my computer in the UK, I received an order from Pennsylvania in the USA. That night, I packaged a shrink-wrapped copy of the book; the next day I sent it in the mail and a few weeks afterwards I received an email saying that the reader had received his order. I find this sequence of events extraordinary.

I had never been to Pennsylvania, and the customer had never before heard of me let alone met me. Yet he read about the book on the website, liked what he read and clicked on a button. This transferred money from his US bank account to my UK bank account, and sent me an email to alert me that I needed to keep my part of the bargain. I then sent the book to him across 3000 miles of sea, and he seems to have greatly enjoyed reading it. Events like these continued to happen over the next few months, and thousands of people around the world are benefiting from these systems of international trade. It all begins with PayPal.

PayPal

PayPal started out as a small American company that let anyone transfer money to anyone else in America. In the UK and Europe we have been used to this kind of service for many years, but for Americans it was incredible that they were not being charged for it. However, PayPal went on to do much more. They allowed these transfers through the Internet and mobile phones. They then expanded to allow transfers between an increasing number of countries (albeit with charges), and they allowed anyone to accept transfers from a credit card.

It costs nothing to get an account through PayPal's website (http://www.paypal.com), and only a little effort to integrate their buttons into your own website. Your website can then sell your book, and the buttons can accept payments. When you start handling a greater number of payments for a larger range of products and you want more professionalism to your site, try going for WorldPay (www.worldpay.com)

Postage

The UK is blessed with the Royal Mail. Sending packages is surprisingly cheap and reliable. Three things are worth noting. First, writing 'Printed Papers' on the package qualifies you for reduced costs. This label is a great help for any publisher. Second, for overseas postage you often have to document the package's content and cost, in case the buyer has to pay customs' tax. Make friends with your post office clerk and they will guide you through this process.

Finally, postage will take up a lot of your time. Initially, making trips to the post office will be a pleasure because it is confirmation that someone somewhere wants your book enough to pay for it. But soon the trips become tiring, and you will wish for someone else to take on this role. This is the time to consider selling your book to a publisher. Traditional publishers will also have the contacts and industry know-how to achieve greater penetration into your target market, and thus will increase the readership of your book (and your financial return in the process).

Selling to another publisher

If your book becomes a success, a larger publisher may be interested in buying it from you. This is great because they will take on many of the tasks that you found tedious, such as marketing and order management. It also means you start from a position of power – the standard contract that they send you becomes a starting point for negotiations, because you have already taken away the risk of publishing an unpopular book (as you are already making regular sales). All that remains is to choose your publisher wisely – each has strengths and weaknesses, and you must make sure that these match your book's needs. As always, research carefully and confer with your mentors.

Is it all worth it?

So, you have written, printed, published, marketed and sold your own book. Are you now rich? Rarely. If you do your job well, you should be able to get some good money for your efforts. Of course, you can get even better money by working in a more traditional job for that same number of hours. If money is your motivation, there are better ways to make it.

On the other hand, being an author is of course a tremendous boost to your CV and hence your upward mobility.

Furthermore, there is something different about money that you earn through your enterprise and innovation. And then, of course, there are the letters from readers who have enjoyed your book. To me, these make it all worthwhile.

REFERENCES

http://www.useit.com/alertbox/9710a.html – an excellent article on tailoring your writing style to suit readers of websites.

Poynter D. *The Self-Publishing Manual.* Santa Barbera, CA: Para Publishing, 2003.

10

HOW TO GET A BOOK PUBLISHED PROFESSIONALLY

Georgina Bentliff

The previous chapter on 'How to publish your own book'
is all about what is known as 'self-publishing' – writing the
book, or the electronic equivalent, you want to write, and
broadcasting the message you want to send. Commercial
publishing is rather different. It is about the publications that
other people – 'the market' – want to read or, in medicine,
more likely want to 'use'. Most people do not read a medical
book because they have a moral duty to know about a subject;
they do so because they need to pass an exam or cope with a
practical hurdle. Always be clear for what purpose you are
writing.

Having a published book to your name is an eye-catching and
relatively unusual item to include in your CV. It suggests that
you can come up with an original idea, have the persistence to
find a publisher, and can deliver in terms of actually getting the
book written or edited. It is unusual, but not unknown, for a
medical student to have written a book. The Crash Course series
from Mosby was initiated by a medical student; so was Hodder
Arnold's One Stop Doc series, and all its authors are students.
Indeed, this very book is an honourable example of a book

conceived and largely written by a medical student. In addition, there are very many medical authors whose first book was a self-assessment text written shortly after success in tackling the MRCP or MRCS (I will tend to talk about publishing your 'book' for simplicity's sake, but this could of course be a website or CD.).

If you want to join this group there are some fundamental steps you will need to take. I will describe these from the point of view of the commissioning editor – the individual with whom you are likely to have most contact, especially when you first approach a publishing house with your big idea.

The commissioning editor may variously be called the 'acquisitions editor', 'the publisher' or simply 'the editor'; the crucial point is that you will be dealing with the individual whose job it is to 'sign' new 'product' for a company and to ensure that what he or she has 'signed' is delivered successfully. Other publishing activities, such as design or marketing, will be done by other people, but your communication with those others will almost always be through the commissioning editor. For this reason, it is important that you get on well with this person; if you find you dislike them from the word go you should probably try a different company!

THE CONCEPT

What is your book going to be about? Publishers often start out by talking to students about the books they have liked and not liked, and the opportunities they see for new publications, so search your own memory for the times you have thought 'If only X existed.' Talk to your friends about what they wish was available. Revision and self-assessment tend to be good bets because you, the student, are going to have a much better idea of what will help your fellow students remember things than your lecturers will.

APPROACHING A PUBLISHER

If you feel you have an idea that is practical and simple (nobody wants unnecessary complications) you will need to choose an appropriate publisher. Almost certainly there will already be some sort of competition for your idea. The publisher of that competitor may be looking for more of the same, but on the whole rival publishers will be more interested, especially if the existing competition is known to be successful.

Some important dos and don'ts in approaching a publisher

Do:

- Choose a publisher with publications of a similar sort already. Are they already publishing books for medical students? Most publishers don't like having a solitary 'orphan' title, as opportunities for marketing it will be much more limited. Are they already publishing self-assessment books at university level and might be interested in moving into medicine? Few publishers will want to do something that is a totally new departure: rather, they would prefer to build on something they have already found to be successful.
- Contact the publisher and ask what form they like a proposal to take. They may well have a standard form to use, or a checklist of items; if they do, you would be very sensible to use it and ensure that all the information needed is made available at the outset.
- If a sample section of the book is required, go for quality not quantity. The publisher will be looking for a flavour of the overall book and your ability as a writer. They will be sharing this material with their advisers (more about 'advisers' later). Bad spelling or grammar can bring reading to a halt in the first paragraph, and it sounds pretty feeble to say 'It was just a first draft', when you should be giving the proposal your best shot.

- Be clear who you are writing for. It is a joke among commissioning editors that proposals arrive from authors who say they are writing for 'the specialist, medical students, and the informed general reader'. Quite clearly each of these three groups requires information at a different level of detail and explanation; one book is not going to satisfy all three, and is consequently unlikely to be appropriate for any of them.
- Be clear why your target audience will buy your book. Will it be to pass a particular exam? Or to get them through a difficult component of their course? And what will it offer in doing so that is not already available?
- Anticipate that your proposal may be changed by the publisher rather than be accepted exactly as originally presented. The commissioning editor may see in your project the germ of something that will be far bigger than your original conception: a single book may become a series; a book on a single topic may be broadened to become a comprehensive textbook. Don't be too proud about sticking to your original idea, but allow yourself to take on board the publisher's ideas. You may of course find you really don't agree with them, but keep an open mind.

Don't

- Waste the publisher's time. If you are approaching more than one publisher at the same time you should tell all concerned. It is very annoying as a commissioning editor to discover that you have put a lot of effort into researching the viability of a proposal only to discover at the last minute you are being forced to bid against another publisher. In these circumstances my response would be that the author is not straightforward and therefore not someone I want to work with anyway.
- Hassle the commissioning editor on a daily basis as to the progress of their research into your proposal. They will be working on a lot of projects at the same time, so getting in touch fortnightly will help to keep your project up the priority list, but anything more than that will give the impression

that you are a pain, and they will not want to pursue the relationship however promising your proposal.

- Rubbish the competition. If it's selling there must be something good about it. Far better to pick out its good and weak points and explain how you can improve on them.
- Get an agent! Novelists have agents but academic authors rarely do, and most publishers will be put off rather than impressed to have an additional person to deal with.

THE PUBLISHER'S PERSPECTIVE

Publishing companies are constantly looking for new ideas. Without new publications their businesses will cease to grow, and ultimately they will fail. They employ commissioning editors to find those new publications, and the commissioning editors are judged by the value of what they commission. Furthermore, they will be considering lots of new projects at the same time, and prioritizing them, and anything ill-defined or overly complicated will not stand a chance. Here are some of the things the commissioning editor will be thinking about when considering your new idea:

- 'Who is this person?' Include a short CV about your medical training and any writing you've done. They will not be interested in where you went to school or what you got in your A levels, but they will want to know which medical school you're at, what year you're in, and how you've been performing in your exams.
- 'On what authority will this person be writing?' Have a co-author or 'editorial adviser' lined up who is both senior and credible.
- 'How big is the market for this book?' The publisher should know, for example, how many medical students there are or how many people take USMLE (United States Medical Licensing Exam) annually, but if you know and say so it's much more impressive. (Do check your facts, though; if you get it wrong the publisher is not going to be impressed.)

- 'How expensive will this publication be to produce?' The elements that cost most are colour printing (even today), line drawings (complicated operative surgery or anatomical can come in at £75 per piece), 'permissions' (payment to use material that has already been published elsewhere), and any software development. If you want to make your project easily affordable go for a single-colour printed book with no illustrations and no material borrowed from elsewhere.
- 'Will this justify our overheads?' Publishing is a labour-intensive business and your project has got to pay for the time of a great many people and still make a profit. The team includes the commissioning editor, the desk editor (the person who will liaise with you during the production process), the copyeditor (the person who reads every word for grammar, spelling, and consistency of fact and style), the production controller (the person who contracts the typesetter and the printer and buys the paper), the proofreader, the indexer, the typesetter, the printer, the marketing executive, several sales reps, the accounts staff, the warehouse staff and the office cleaners.
- 'What will be the overall turnover and profit from this project?' A £9.99 book that could sell 10 000 copies is worth considering, as is £99 book that could sell 1000 copies, but a £9.99 book that is unlikely to sell more than 2000 copies is hardly going to be worth getting out of bed for, unless the publisher has minimal overheads.

Once the commissioning editor is reassured that you and your project are worth considering they are likely to proceed as follows. He or she will get 'market feedback' from a cross-section of people ('advisers') who the publisher believes are representative of the project's target market. In the case of a publication for medical students, they will show your proposal and sample material to lecturers and to students, and ask them whether it is relevant to their courses and whether they think they would buy it, were it available. This means quite a few unknown people (this sort of reviewing is usually done anonymously) will get to know about your idea; you may feel uncomfortable about this, and of course those reviewers could steal off to another publisher and present it as their idea, but publishers are great respecters of copyright as it is entirely in their interests to be so.

The publisher will also get a proper estimate of production costs, so a sound projection of profit and loss can be made. If the production costs are compatible with estimated turnover and the response from advisers is positive (though they will often recommend improvements) the commissioning editor will then be ready to accept your proposal, but it is very rare that your commissioning editor can make a unilateral decision to do so. Even in relatively small companies the decision will be a joint one involving marketing and sales people, and will generally involve a formal committee to which your proposal will be presented. Only if the marketing and sales people agree with estimated sales and the use of overhead will your project be formally accepted by the publishing company.

WHAT TO ASK YOUR COMMISSIONING EDITOR ONCE YOUR PROJECT HAS BEEN ACCEPTED

The euphoria of having your proposal accepted should not drive out practical considerations, and before you sign a formal Publisher's Agreement you would be wise to get clear answers to the following:

- How many copies do you expect to sell?
- How many copies will you print to begin with?
- How will you price my book?
- How long will it take you to publish it once I have sent you the manuscript? (Six months is quite good going for most book publishers, so don't assume it will be out in a couple of weeks.)
- Can you show me a marketing plan for my book?

- How will you market my book *after* publication? (The big marketing push is always before publication. Books that are no longer 'new' can have a hard time of it.)
- How will you sell my book overseas?
- Do you have a team of sales reps who call on bookshops? In which countries?
- Do you have a team of sales reps who call on medical schools? In which countries? Will they carry my book?
- What medical conferences do you attend regularly that will be relevant to my book?

You may get answers you do not want to hear, but at least there will be no false assumptions and cause for falling out later on. For example, you may think pricing your book at £29.99 will be the kiss of death. Discuss it with the publisher. If they are convinced they are right you can still withdraw the project, but the chances are that another publisher will think the same on the basis of similar production costs and similar sales experience.

WHAT TO EXPECT IN YOUR PUBLISHER'S AGREEMENT

Once your project has been accepted for publication your commissioning editor will send you a formal Publisher's Agreement setting out the terms under which publication will take place. This is a legal document, but I suggest that you do not get a lawyer friend whose usual work is, say, conveyancing to advise you on it. Your publisher will probably tell you to get lost before you've raised half the questions your lawyer friend has listed, especially if this well-meaning individual gets badly exercised about TV rights. If you want sound advice based on long experience in academic publishing, join the Society of Authors' and get them to look at it. They will immediately be able to reassure you what is standard across publishers and what is potentially problematic.

Don't, on the other hand, sign your Agreement without even reading it, as no one can have much sympathy with you later if you've agreed to something unfair or unrealistic without even checking. Here are some important things to look for:

● Will you keep copyright or be handing it over to the publisher? To make publishing your book worthwhile you will need to grant your publisher 'exclusive licence' to publish it, at least in the form agreed (you may want to hang on to electronic rights or publishing rights in one particular country, for example), but it is always best for you if you can retain ownership of your copyright.

● Is the deadline for completing the work realistic? If you don't meet the deadline the publisher will have the right to cancel the Agreement, and though this is unlikely to happen unless you are literally years late, it is much better not to take the risk.

● Is the extent of the book (numbers of words and illustrations) listed in the Agreement realistic? Again, the publisher will have the right to refuse your manuscript if it does not conform to what has been agreed, so be sure that you are not signing up to something that does not conform to your expectations.

● Who is going to be producing the index? Almost all publishers now commission an index from a professional indexer at their own expense, but they may be expecting you to compile it yourself. Don't let yourself in for a nasty surprise later.

● How many complimentary (gratis) copies will you get? If you are the sole author, it really doesn't make much difference to the publisher if you receive ten rather than five gratis copies, so it's always worth trying to secure a few extra at this early stage.

● What royalty are you being offered? The standard in academic publishing would currently be 10 per cent of 'net sales receipts'. The latter is a very important distinction from 'published price'. Fiction authors, for example, will generally get a lower royalty but it will be based on 'published price'. That is, if their book is priced at £9.99 they will receive x per cent of £9.99 for every copy sold, no matter what the publisher is paid for it. In academic publishing it will depend on the route by which your book is sold. If the publisher sells your book direct to the customer for its full price of £9.99, you will receive 99p for that copy. If it sells through a bookshop the publisher will only receive £7 at most for it, so you will receive 70p, that is, 10 per cent of the publisher's net receipts after the bookseller has taken their cut. For your first book you will be very lucky to negotiate anything higher than 10 per cent, and it may well be that the 'riskiness' of the venture requires a considerably lower royalty, at least at the outset. If that is the case, argue for a rising royalty so that once your publication is established (e.g. after 2000 copies have sold) you will be getting a percentage that is close to standard.

● What proportion of any sales of rights are you being offered? The most likely rights deals involving your book will not relate to TV but to translation rights. Your book might, for example, be published by a Mexican publisher in Spanish. It is standard to share what the foreign-language publisher pays 50:50 with your principal publisher.

There is one element of the standard agreement with which many authors have a problem. This relates to indemnifying the publisher for aspects of your writing over which the publisher has little control: plagiarism, libel and errors of fact. The publisher will generally be insured against these eventualities, but only you will know if you are ripping off someone else's work or telling untruths about someone, and the reason that the publisher has trusted you to write the book is that you should know what facts are correct. If you are very unhappy about agreeing to indemnify the publisher you may find some modifications can be introduced, but it is up to you to write a squeaky-clean book.

THE PUBLISHING PROCESS

Once you have completed and submitted your manuscript you can expect a process along the following lines.

Manuscript assessment

The publisher will want to have a good look at what you've submitted to ensure it conforms with expectations in terms of content and extent. This may involve having it reviewed by further 'advisers', who may suggest additional changes. Check with your commissioning editor ahead of time to see whether this is going to happen, again so that there are no surprises.

Copyediting

If all is in order, your manuscript and illustrations will be handed to a copyeditor, who will read every word and correct inconsistencies in spelling, grammar and style. If references are missing or there are contradictions in the text, for example, the copyeditor will raise questions for you to answer. It is very unusual for there to be no such questions, so don't be defensive when the copyeditor contacts you. Copyediting is generally the most time-consuming element in the whole production process: by answering queries quickly you will be able to prevent unnecessary delays.

Most copyediting is now done on screen and the copyeditor adds codes to your manuscript that will be translated into levels of heading (the hierarchy of headings that will give your manuscript a lot of its structure), layout of tables and refer- ences, and 'special features' such as boxes of key points. Don't spend a lot of time formatting your manuscript before you hand it over, as all the formatting will be stripped out by the copyeditor and an entirely new set of codes introduced.

Illustration

If your project includes line drawings that need to be specially drawn, a medical artist will be commissioned to produce these while copyediting is in progress. You should be given an opportunity to check the drawings before page proofs are made up, provided that publication is not on a very tight schedule.

Typesetting

The copyedited text, together with any illustrations (line drawings plus digitized photographs), will be sent to a typesetter, who will use the basic material to form 'printed' pages to conform to an agreed design. This may be a standard design that the publisher regularly uses, or something special for your project. Ask in advance so that you know what to expect.

Proofreading

The page proofs produced by the typesetter will need to be thoroughly checked, though the electronic manuscript has eliminated a lot of the crazy typographical errors that old-fashioned keying used to introduce. Has material been left out? Are your illustrations the right way up? Are they in the right place? Almost always a professional proofreader will also be checking the proofs against your original manuscript, so you can concentrate on broad-brush issues rather than re-reading word for word. What you will not be able to do at this relatively late stage is rewrite whole sections because seeing them in print makes you feel suddenly unhappy with them. Neither can you add significant amounts of new material. Your Agreement may well say that if you make lots of corrections because of your own change of heart you will have to carry the additional cost.

Indexing

This takes place at the same time as proofreading and is generally done by a professional indexer. It is helpful to agree with your commissioning editor what sort of index your book needs: should it be very detailed, or just include basic entries? Is there another book you can cite that has an index that you would like yours to resemble? You will generally be given a chance to see the index before it is typeset.

Advance copies

Following that, you can expect to see your first copies of the book, hot off the press and looking alarmingly public and open to criticism. Don't open your book and immediately look for errors; savour having it for a few days. Make sure you thank your publisher for sending the copies – you would be surprised how many authors don't!

11

HOW TO MAKE GREAT PRESENTATIONS

Riaz Agha

Throughout medical school and your clinical career you will be making presentations. Indeed, being able to consistently make great presentations to audience after audience can have a tremendous impact on your future career. Great presentations not only get you good marks but also get you noticed. Whenever you produce a significant body of work, always try and see if you can present it at either local departmental, regional, national or international level.

When preparing to make a presentation, remember that busy people will be coming to hear you speak: while presenting, you have mastery over their visual and auditory environment as well as their precious time. This is a special opportunity, and you must make the most if it and do your best. Try to captivate and interest your audience, and keep this in mind when preparing and delivering your presentation. Remember, no matter how good your content, if its delivery is poor the content will become irrelevant and no-one will be interested.

Presentations can be broken up into two components – public speaking and visual aids (e.g. PowerPoint, overhead projector, etc.). Both are considered in detail in this chapter, and both need to be well prepared and thought out for a great presentation. The skills of good public speaking will also help when giving speeches, where visual aids may not be present/required.

PUBLIC SPEAKING

The very thought of speaking to a large audience about anything is daunting, and for some people even terrifying. However, everyone improves with practice, and there are many things you can do to improve your performance. Good public speaking consists of two elements, the preparation and the performance. Thorough preparation is the surest way of building your confidence, and this in turn will affect your performance.

Preparation

Thorough preparation consists of asking the pertinent questions:

- What is the aim of the presentation? What message do you want your audience to take away?
- What is your remit? What is the range of content you are supposed to cover?
- Why you? Do you have special knowledge in this area?
- Who is coming? This will help you pitch your content appropriately.
- How much time will you have?
- Where will it take place? What will the ambience and facilities be like? This will also help you set the appropriate typeface for the text on your visual aids.
- What audiovisual facilities will be available (e.g. PowerPoint or overhead projector only?), and will you be allowed to use a CD or will only floppy disks be accepted?
- How many people are coming? Will it be a small room or a large conference hall?
- Be sure you know how to get there.

Have a very clear idea about what message you want to deliver and what information you want to transfer. You then need to gather this information through a process of research. For example, if you have been asked to give a talk on 'myocardial infarction (MI) management', you would start your research by reading a section in a textbook on MI management, followed by the latest journal review articles on the subject, consulting with others, and so on. Great presenters always know their subject matter inside out, so they can give a confident presentation and are easily able to handle questions at the end. If you are doing a presentation based on a report or essay you have written, read it through several times over until you can provide a summary of each section's points almost from memory. This will minimize the chances of losing your train of thought during the presentation.

Once you have gathered the information you need through your research, read it all through and decide on the main points. It is often helpful to create a Microsoft Word file of the main sections of the presentation and the main points you want to make in each. You can then cut and paste these sections into Microsoft PowerPoint and adjust the style and so on. Building up the content of your presentation in Word first allows you to see an overview of your talk and set about structuring your presentation, without having to worry about moving things from one slide to another in PowerPoint. Whichever program you are working in, don't forget to save your work regularly and create a backup which you can update as you go along.

Always construct your presentations with an introduction, a middle and a conclusion: this follows the format of the old adage, 'tell them what you are going to tell them, tell them, and then tell them what you have told them'.

Introduction

At the very start, remember to introduce yourself, your position and your institution (if you are at a conference, for example). If there is a Chairman, thank them first; always try and be as professional as possible while at the same time not appearing overly pedantic or rigid. You need to follow this with an outline of what you are going to talk about: this will inform the audience of the boundaries of your talk and its aims. If you want to grab people's attention and truly influence them, you have to interest them right from the start. A good technique is to ask the question you ultimately hope to answer. This challenges listeners and shows that you hope to structure your presentation around a central question they can refer to; it also states clearly what your presentation is all about. Other techniques include giving a famous quotation, or even telling a short story.

Middle

The main bulk of your presentation should consist of a set of key points, each of which you expand upon by presenting data, results or arguments to support a particular position. Your intention should to be to have no more than three to five bullet points per slide (with more important points in larger text): any more than this and you risk overwhelming your audience, as people can only hold a certain number of details in their mind while following your overall logic. The details that follow each point can be built up in your Word document, and it is this that you can read over and over again to make sure that you know your material well. Each slide should provide one to two minutes of material to talk about at most (the audience can get very frustrated if you take ages over each slide: steady progress in your slide transitions helps to relieve some of this tension).

It's also a good idea to number your points, as this way the audience knows how much material you have left and how you are progressing. Take the time to build up complex arguments, always make your points flow logically from one to another, make it easy for people to follow your arguments, and remember to stick to the main points. When preparing your presentation, imagine yourself in the audience: would you get bored if the speaker went through all that detail? How could it be shortened to give it greater impact? Would you get confused if that process was explained in that way? Try and use your slides to provide yourself with key words and cues for you to discuss rather than simply for the audience to read. This also makes you more non-committal, so if your audience turns out to be more knowledgeable than you expected you can adjust accordingly.

Try to use real-life case histories to explain some of your points if possible: this fires the imagination of the audience and gets them thinking and re-engaged with the presentation.

Audiences respond well to changes in visual material, so use colourful photos, diagrams, graphs and flowcharts rather than text when you can. For more complex flowcharts, diagrams or graphs, make sure people know where to start and try and guide them through as you speak, using a laser pen (avoid making circular motions with the laser: keep it steady and draw smoothly).

Conclusion

Always finish with a definitive conclusion: never say 'erm, that's it really'. This is the classic phrase people use and it sounds awful. It's always good to inform the audience that you are concluding, rather than taking them by surprise: for example, you could say, 'To conclude, it's worth stating these four points. . . .' This provides the 'endgame' signal to your audience and focuses their attention once more. Try and vary your language as much as possible, expressing the same points slightly differently, for example; this makes people think you haven't said the same thing before, and at the same time reinforces the message. The conclusion should not result in any diversions or in your being sidetracked. Each point should be the conclusion of something you discussed in more detail earlier. It should, in essence, bring you full circle, and you may want to repeat the question you stated in the introduction. There is usually no point in having a references slide follow the conclusions: it is better to put them in as footnotes as you go along (after all, who is going to stare at them for 2 minutes, reading them?).

Final rehearsal

At the end of this process you should have created a neat set of concise notes that you can use to rehearse prior to the delivery of your presentation. Once you know your core material inside out, these notes can be exchanged for a printout of your slides, with any additional points that do not appear on the slides written in the margins. You need to convert them from a 'written' style to one that is going to be spoken out loud. The worst – and unfortunately one of the most common – mistake is for presenters to read out exactly what it says on their slides. Remember to make the typeface of the text appropriate to the occasion and the size of the room, and to avoid clutter on your slides.

Your audiovisual aids should now all be prepared (see PowerPoint section) and you are ready to rehearse your presentation as you will give it. Keep doing this until you reach a point where you hardly need to look at your slides: one point flows logically on to the next. It is helpful to practise out loud and to time yourself till you finish at about 80% of the allotted time – the actual performance always takes more time. In any case, audiences always forgive someone for finishing early, and Chairmen will be happy you got them back on schedule. If you go over the allotted time in practice, can you shave off extra words or unnecessary points to get the time down (remember, a simple diagram or flowchart can save a lot of time in place of a slide of prose).

Rehearsing your speech over and over again should not result in monotony in your delivery or a lack of spontaneity: as George Bernard Shaw, the Nobel Prize-winning dramatist and literary critic, once remarked: 'I am the most spontaneous speaker in the world because every word, every gesture and every retort has been carefully rehearsed'. So practise in front of family, friends, or on your own; run through your content and master the timing and the slide transitions.

If requested, and if appropriate, it might be worth printing handouts of your slides for your audience (six slides per page is usually sufficient). Of course, for larger audiences this may be inappropriate, and people often spend a disproportionate amount of time looking at handouts they are given – which in any case should always mirror the presented slides – and thus they pay less attention to you. If you expect your audience to annotate your handouts and think they would appreciate the opportunity to do this, then give them out beforehand; if not, give them out at the end of your talk. Remember to pack a backup CD or floppy disk of your presentation, and you may even take a backup acetate version of your PowerPoint slides for very important presentations. If you can't fit your presentation on a single floppy, try compressing the images in Adobe Photoshop; avoid the 'pack and go' feature in PowerPoint (where the presentation is compressed on to a set of floppy disks): it's just too risky to use for something so important. It's a good idea to email the final presentation to yourself: if your CD or floppy disk don't work or disappear on the day for some reason, then you may be able to download it and still use your PowerPoint version rather than resort to acetates.

In cases where both PowerPoint and OHP facilities are provided it might be worth leaving an acetate of the overall structure of your talk on the OHP to which people can refer as you go through the PowerPoint slides. Also, have a good think about what you will wear on the day, what kind of meeting it is, and who will be coming: would you feel comfortable talking to people in those clothes? In general, it's better to be more professional, as you can always dress down and leave yourself with more options. Remember, you are presenting your content and yourself as an individual, and people need to think you are respectable and believable. Don't forget to pack your laser pen, and if you are presenting at a conference always pack a few business cards to distribute to interested parties after the presentation.

On the day itself

A good breakfast is often underrated these days, but it all goes towards being 'on the ball' and minimizing any distractions during your presentation. Always take your mobile phone and know who to contact in case you are running late (turn it off before you start, of course). Arrive early, liaise with the organizers and load up your presentation: does it work? are the edges cut off? have the figures loaded? and, so on. Also, transfer your presentation on to the hard drive of the laptop you will be using: this will prevent any pauses during slide transition, as the CD or floppy is accessed before pictures are shown.

If you bring your own laptop, don't turn it on until after you have connected it to the data projector. You may need to load the drivers for a plug-and-play monitor or your laptop and the data projector won't communicate (do this from the 'add new hardware wizard' icon in the 'control panel'). Movies may run on your laptop screen but not in the projected image. To get around this, go to the 'control panel', choose 'appearance and themes', then 'display', and then select the 'settings' tab, click on 'advanced' and then select the 'displays' tab. You will see your laptop monitor and the data projector labelled 1 and 2, respectively; you need to select the data projector as the primary display and the laptop as the secondary. Use your remaining time to settle your nerves, drink some coffee to increase your alertness, and ensure you keep a bottle of water with you to prevent a dry mouth.

Performance

A great performance starts in the mind: you need to feel that what you have to say is relevant, of fundamental interest to the audience, and that you are the best person to deliver it. You must resolve this in your own mind and have the self-belief to pull it off with confidence. The biggest guarantee of this self-belief is thorough preparation.

In any presentation we have to project an image of ourselves which is often very different from when we have a regular conversation with someone, and at the same time we must maintain our personal touch or people won't believe us.

During the presentation:

● Don't rush because you are nervous. You will end up with your audience struggling to catch up and, as a result, they may lose interest. Set a relaxed and balanced pace with which you are comfortable. Slow down your breathing and don't get worked up.
● Don't speak as you inhale: this will make you sound nervous and this will translate to your audience; it will also affect the clarity of your speech.

- Make sure each point is made clearly and that the important points are made the most forcefully, with clarity, diction and projection. Remember to vary your tone, pace and volume.

- Don't present your talk to the projector or screen. Avoid looking backwards and constantly moving your head back and forth to read off your slides; this gives the impression you didn't prepare thoroughly (the same goes for reading from your notes, as this leads to monotony as well). If anything, look at the screen of the laptop in front of you. You can also use the 'notes' facility when constructing your presentation, to allow you to see the extra things you want to say on the laptop screen (which aren't projected for the audience to see).

- Keep looking at your audience even when the slides change, move on to the next topic and keep things moving; this gives an air of professionalism and the audience will see it (it's also more 'cool').

- Resist the temptation to pace up and down in front of the screen like a caged tiger.

- Avoid cracking obvious jokes – the audience may not laugh and you will look like a complete clown. Use subtle humour if you must – it's less risky.

- Be aware of your gestures and hand movements: try to make them proportionate to the point you are trying to make, and avoid swinging your arms aimlessly.

- Be aware of your posture: don't lean on anything or turn your back to the audience in an arrogant or patronizing manner (remember, you are privileged to be presenting – it is not a right).

- Be aware of your position in relation to the projector screen, the projector and the audience: don't stand where your shadow will cover the screen.

- Be aware of the quality of output from your microphone: watch for any feedback and beware of losing the microphone when you turn your head.

- Don't hold any notes in your hands while giving your presentation: not only can this be distracting for the audience, it also prevents you from using your hands to communicate.

- Try to pause at appropriate moments to allow the audience to take in your last point.
- Make sure you survey the entire audience and don't just stare straight ahead. Make as much eye contact and try to engage your audience as much as possible.
- Try to make every member of the audience feel special. When you meet someone's eyes briefly, give them your full attention. Keep this up, and eventually most people think they were specially focused on.
- Anticipate distractions such as mobile phones or late arrivals and learn to ignore them.

The performance is the most nerve-racking part of the process, and this is where your thorough preparation pays off. Don't expect perfection too soon: observe how other people give presentations, look at their strengths and weaknesses, and learn from them. Everyone improves their public speaking skills with practice, and you will too; it will get easier and more enjoyable with time.

Answering questions

Questions can be a good sign: no-one asks questions of a boring speaker (because they weren't listening in the first place!). Always attempt to predict the questions that may be asked during your preparation. Make sure you know the issues regarding your content, as well as the content itself. A classic error is to go off at a tangent into something of interest to yourself, instead of answering actual questions. Don't lose sight of the question: hold it in your mind and refer back to it, if possible, at the end of your answer. Avoid getting sidetracked and deal with each question fully and succinctly. Remember to state your position on an issue at the beginning and at the end. If you don't have all the information to answer the question, say so: your audience will appreciate that you view the situation as complex and not straightforward. Try to give the questioner the feeling that they learnt something and that they have come away with the information or advice they were looking for.

POWERPOINT

For the purposes of this section a certain amount of knowledge is assumed. Readers are referred to the book *PowerPoint for Dummies* to build their basic knowledge.

Useful shortcuts

Ctrl + s   = Save file

Ctrl + z   = Undo previous steps (up to 20 steps)

Ctrl + a   = Select all

Ctrl + c   = Copies selection

Ctrl + x   = Cut text

Ctrl + v   = Paste text

Ctrl + f   = Find word in text

Ctrl + b   = Bolds selection

Ctrl + i   = Italicizes selection

Shift + F3   = Toggle capitals on/off

Slide Layout (from the 'format' menu)

You are in complete control of the organization of each slide, but initially you need a template to work with. The Slide Layout option provides these templates, some being for text only and some having space for a diagram.

Slide Master (from the 'View' menu, click on 'Master' and then 'Slide Master')

Although your slides may have different layouts, they can still have a consistent overall feel. Changes you make in the Slide Master will apply to every slide.

Slide transitions

Don't have text flying in from different angles – in fact, avoid animations altogether if you can: audiences find them very irritating and it can give them an awful headache. Your slide transitions should be subtle and uniform and should be silent (no screeching sounds please).

Rehearse Timings (from the 'Slide Show' menu)

This setting allows you to practise your presentation and see how long you spend on each slide, as well as how long the entire presentation takes. You can also pause the clock when you need to make minor adjustments to your slides as you go along.

Drawing – diagrams and flowcharts (from the 'View' menu, select 'Toolbars' and check 'Drawing')

Click on 'AutoShapes' on the left side of the drawing toolbar. This reveals a range of shapes that you can select and place on the slide and subsequently resize. Add some colour by selecting the paint icon on the drawing toolbar and selecting the colour you want. You can also change the colour of the border by selecting the paintbrush. You can place text boxes within or around your shapes by clicking on the 'text box' icon in the 'drawing' toolbar.

Guides and grids (from the 'View' menu)

Guides and grids help to keep the presentation consistent, for example if you want to line up a picture in the same place on successive slides. The *guide* lines will be the same across your entire presentation (if you change them on one slide, they will change for all slides). You can, however, also change guide lines on an individual slide. You can move the guide lines by dragging them with the left mouse button. When you move pictures or shapes about on a screen, they move according to the *grid*: this is manifest by the jagged movements of the shape: the wider apart the grid lines, the more jagged these movements will be. Sometimes you may want to place your shapes, diagrams or photos more precisely: for this you need to break free from the grid. Press and hold down the 'Alt' key while dragging the shape around the screen. If you want to move the shape in a straight line along x- or y-axes, press and hold the 'Shift' key together with the 'Alt' key (e.g. when you want 'before' and 'after' photos to line up precisely).

Connectors (from the 'Drawing' toolbar and 'Autoshapes' menu)

If you are making a flowchart, using connectors can save huge amounts of time. If you create two text boxes and have a connector between them, no matter where you move the boxes they will stay connected.

Grouping (Shift-select all shapes and then press right click)

If you press Shift and then click on all your shapes, then right-click, select 'grouping' and then click on 'group', you will have grouped the shapes together and they can all be enlarged, moved and rotated simultaneously and to the same degree.

Importing charts from Microsoft Excel

Make all the formatting changes to the chart before pasting it onto your PowerPoint slide – you will always have more editing options in Excel itself. Pasting a chart into PowerPoint can greatly increase the size of your file, because the chart is not just a picture but also all of the tagged data – essentially you are pasting the entire Excel file. To get around this, instead of pasting a chart normally, go to the 'Edit' menu and click on 'Paste special', then select 'Picture (Enhanced Metafile)'. Then right-click on the chart and select 'Grouping' and 'Ungroup'. You have now pasted just the chart, which you can resize and move normally without the excess file size.

Images from Adobe Photoshop

Images can greatly increase the size of a presentation, so you need to cut them down to size. In Adobe Photoshop, try cropping the image and getting rid of unnecessary parts or borders. Another method is to go to the 'File' menu and select 'Save for Web': a new window will pop up where you can alter the resolution of your picture. Select 'Constrain proportions' (to maintain the width/height relationships of the image) and then change the resolution to a lower number, e.g. if width is 3200 change it to 1000 – the height will change automatically in proportion. You can see what the new file size is in the bottom left corner of your screen. You can alter the JPEG compressions setting when you save your file: this will sacrifice image quality in exchange for a smaller file. However, all pictures will be 72 dpi by default if you do this, so if you don't want to lose image quality (e.g. for poster presentations), its better to use the 'Image size' option in the Photoshop Image menu. Such tools are very important when you have too many images to fit on a floppy and the laptop doesn't have a CD-ROM drive.

How to do batch conversions

If you need to convert a large number of picture files in a PowerPoint presentation to a smaller size all in one go, use IrfanView, a free program which you can download from http://www.irfanview.com. Once installed:

- Open the PowerPoint file and save it to the desktop as a web page (e.g. call the file 'test').
- Open IrfanView and select 'File' and then 'Batch conversion/rename'.
- Then select the folder for 'Test_files' (located on the desktop as well).
- Click on 'Add all'.
- Under 'Output directory', click on 'Browse' and select 'test_files'.
- Under 'Work as' select 'Batch conversion'.
- Check the box for 'Use advanced options' and click on 'Set advanced options'.
- Check 'Resize' and click on 'Set new size as a percentage of the original'.
- Check 'Use Resample function (better quality)' and then press 'OK'.

- Under 'Output format' it will usually say JPEG; you can change this to whatever output format you want for the files you have selected.
- Click on 'Start' and then on 'Exit'.
- Start PowerPoint and then open the 'test' web page file and save it as a PowerPoint file.

You have now taken a presentation full of large picture files and reduced their size and hence that of the whole presentation file all in one go. You can of course choose to reduce the size of a certain group of files (not all of them), and there are a number of other options in the program that you can explore.

Other points

- Don't use green or red text, as it's very difficult to see and some men are colour-blind.
- Don't feel you have to use bullet points in every slide.
- Use good graphics and simple coloured diagrams or flow-charts to explain concepts where possible.

POSTER PRESENTATIONS

In general, the preparation and performance components of poster presentations are the same as for oral presentations. However, crucially, you must find out:

- How big the posters should be.
- Should your poster design be portrait or landscape?
- Your poster should allow a passer-by to learn the main points in less than a minute.
- It should be readable from a distance of 1–2 metres (a typeface of 24 or 30 point should suffice, but make the main points larger and references smaller).
- Use lower case rather than capitals because blocks of text in capitals are harder to read.
- Avoid green or red writing as with oral presentations, and use no more than three different colours.

- Avoid three-dimensional text as it's harder to read at a distance.
- Ensure people know where to start and how to follow your poster: use arrows to guide them if necessary.
- Don't forget to include your full name, email address and institutional details on your poster.
- Check and re-check your poster for legibility and errors.
- It is helpful to laminate your poster: this will prevent it creasing up or getting damaged in your poster tube or when you hang it up.
- If possible, take some full-text copies of your paper, a handout or a list of references (all of which should contain your contact details) which you can place in a plastic pocket and hang up beside your poster.
- Arrive early and leave plenty of time to set up.
- Bring a pack of business cards.

FURTHER READING

Lowe L. *PowerPoint 2003 for Dummies*. Foster City, CA: IDG Press, 2003.

HOW TO MAKE
SUCCESSFUL JOB
APPLICATIONS

12

HOW TO BUILD A WINNING CV

Carole Hjelm

A CV is a sales tool where you are the product (a self-marketing tool): its most important role is to inspire the reader's interest in you and get you an interview for the job you are applying for. The scope of such jobs varies with time: as a student, you may be applying for a retail job to cover your bills, or applying for funding for that elective; in many cases matching to first post-graduation jobs is carried out by CV application. It goes without saying that in each of these three examples the CV would have a different focus.

Medical CVs differ from those used for any other type of job search, with the exception of academic posts, in that there is no defined length (two pages being the standard length in the UK and one page in the USA) and they should contain a career plan/objective but rarely a personal statement.

POINTS TO REMEMBER

● A CV has only a few seconds to make an impact, and probably gets a 30-second scan before being selected for more detailed reading (or not). You need to ensure that your CV has the best chance of being read in detail and ending up in the 'must interview' pile.

- The first impression a reader gets from your CV is its neatness and layout. Always try to have a greater margin at the bottom of the page, with left-aligned script, as this is probably the most pleasing to the eye.
- Paper quality matters! Use bright white, A4 100 gsm paper so your CV looks different. Cheap paper suggests you don't really care (imagine turning up to an interview in shorts and a vest).
- Make sure your CV is printed with a laser printer to give your text that sharp and clean feel (and they won't smudge).
- Try using 10-point Century Gothic font – it's very clear and easy to read, and again will make your CV standout. If you don't like the look of it, try 12-point Times New Roman.
- It's best to avoid underlining – it can make the CV look old-fashioned.
- Balance the white space by checking the CV on page review first. This is an excellent way to see how crowded or spaced out the text is. If it looks unbalanced, then change the layout. A CV laid out in a pleasing manner with clear organization has a better chance of being selected for reading in more detail.
- Take care with spelling – as well as using spell-check, have someone check the whole document for typographic errors. Taking part in a 'full shit rota' (full shift rota), despite being true, will not endear you to consultants! Poor spelling and typos say that you pay no attention to detail, are lazy, don't really want the job and don't care if you fail. This is probably not true, but don't create that impression.
- Style of writing is personal and tells the reader a lot about you. It is better to use positive action words rather than passive ones, for example the use of the past tense indicates that this is something that the writer has completed, not just taken part in. This gives the impression of someone who is dynamic and decisive. A flamboyant style reflects a confident, outgoing person (who most people would like to work with); dense detail typed in a

tiny font with lots of punctuation betrays a more obsessive personality.

● Finally, remember to keep it short and simple – both the CV and the sentences/statements in it. The selector can always ask questions at interview, so there is no need to put them to sleep reading your CV.

SO, WHAT SHOULD A MEDICAL CV CONTAIN?

The current fashion in CV writing is that the first page should not be headed Curriculum Vitae. However, when applying for junior doctor posts and above, there should be a cover page indicating that this is the CV of Dr X, applying for whatever post, in whichever specialty, at Anywhere Hospital, with the following job reference number. This allows medical staffing personnel to collect all applications for the same post together with little effort on their part, and ensures that your application ends up being read by the right people. If the application has a pro forma for the required CV it is obvious that you should follow that and the instructions. Many Foundation School applications are by CV, which have various pro formae, outlined on their websites around the time of application.

All CVs should provide *personal details*, i.e. name, contact information, including a telephone number and email address, as the first information. It is also a good idea to have your name as a footer on every page, in case some sheets become separated after submission of the CV; remember to number the pages too. Telephone voicemail messages and email addresses should be suitably professional – that fun address or voice message will not do if you are job hunting. Date of birth, gender and nationality should not be placed before the contact information. After registration your GMC number and medical defence number are useful additions to this area of your CV. Photographs are not expected in a UK CV.

Your marital status and number of dependents are entirely your own business and you don't have to disclose this information on a CV.

What next? Now we are in the region of the CV that requires dates. Should they be chronological or reverse chronological order? Unless there are instructions given, the choice is yours. For every consultant who likes a chronological order of dates, there will be one who prefers reverse chronological order. The key is consistency: once you have chosen the order of dates in the first section, this should be adhered to for the rest of the CV. It is not essential to put the months you started and finished a job/school, but the total number of weeks/months in the post may be useful. The other area of consistence for dates is left- or right-aligned? Again the choice is yours, but once made, it should be adhered to.

During your years at university it makes sense to have your *Education/qualifications* as the next section. The MBBS section can be subdivided to include special study modules, exam results, prizes and awards, elective and mini-electives. This can then be followed by *Work experience* – subdivided into relevant and non-relevant – *Extracurricular activities*, *Interests* and finally *Referees*. Once you have started your first post-graduation rotation, this should be presented before your education as your *Current post*.

When applying for jobs just after starting the second rotation the title could be changed to *Pre-registration experience*, to include relevant information about your first post. This tactic cannot be used after registration, when the current post should be on the first page proper of the CV. Medical CVs are unusual in that they include a *Career plan* – at undergraduate level this can be short and general, but later on the statement enables the reader to understand where you are in your career, the relevance of this post and whether you are on track. There is no fixed place for this in the CV, but it is often found after *Education* or *Current post*.

EDUCATION/QUALIFICATIONS

While at university you may include your GCSEs on your CV, but once you have graduated this is less relevant. Don't list all 10 GCSEs – a short summary of 10 GCSEs and the total number of A*, As, Bs, etc., will suffice. Your A-levels should be presented on a single line with the grades in brackets. Don't forget to include that you are studying for your MBBS. For mature students and graduate-entry students GCSEs and A-levels are less relevant.

For your MBBS, include brief details of *Special study modules*, *Research topics* and your *Elective* when you have completed them. Any publications resulting from your work should also be listed in a subsection titled *Publications* within the MBBS section. As you gain more publications through medical school, this should become a separate section inserted between 'career plan' and 'work experience'. This section should be separated under the subheadings *Books*, *Peer-reviewed scientific papers*, *Editorials*, *Abstracts*, *Articles* (in lay media) and *Letters*. You should follow the same formula for *Audits* and *Presentations*. A *Research in progress* section should also be put in if you have got started on something. Any *prizes* and *awards* should also be listed, with a short description of what they were for. You will know – and hopefully consultants linked to the medical school will know – but outside this area the prizes/awards could be for anything. This section will take up a major part of your early CVs. If you intercalate a BSc, this can be entered within the MBBS section; the research project should at least be named in this section, even if you choose to say more about it in an area dedicated to research.

CAREER PLAN

Not only does including this give you the opportunity to explain briefly where you see your medical career progressing, it also allows you to explain why you have applied for this post and helps you to be able to answer the interview question 'Why have you applied for this job?' Most undergraduates have some feeling for what they don't want to do, for example medicine or surgery.

Later in medical school, and as a junior doctor between the *Career plan* and *Work experience* sections, you would place the following: *Research in progress, Audits, Publications, Presentations, Teaching* (e.g. medical students) and Management (e.g. being President of a Student Association or the Junior Doctor's Mess).

WORK EXPERIENCE

In an undergraduate CV this can be split into relevant and other experience. Work done to 'get you into medical school' should not be included in this unless you have continued it while at medical school. For non-medically related work it is best to highlight what you gained from it that will help you be a better doctor. For example, retail work has given you lots of experience communicating with the general public while working in a team. Once qualified, then obviously more information on medical skills is included. Medical skills and specialty experience can be summarized by saying, for example, *x* months of *y* specialty, in list format with the relevant headings.

EXTRACURRICULAR ACTIVITIES

These show the reader that you have been involved in medical school life. If for any reason you have been unable to get involved, include an alternative section headed *Other activities*. This can include work done for the local community, even if it was voluntary. Both these sections can be subdivided into teaching, organizational, sports and community.

INTERESTS

These are personal: you may play a sport for fun as well as representing your college team. Travelling is great, but say where, especially if it is somewhere different. Other general interests include reading, cooking, films and theatre. Don't be vague, give examples of what you read, cook or watch; this makes it much more personal and interesting. However, whatever you do, don't lie. This is one area of the CV that will catch a reader's attention – they may even be looking forward to talking to you about your collection of outer-Mongolian nose flutes, so when you fumble around trying to talk sense they will 'rumble' you, and this will cast doubt on your entire CV. It is better to have only a couple of things that you can talk enthusiastically about, rather than a list of unusual hobbies about which you know next to nothing. Also, don't just list your interests: demonstrate how they developed specific skills and qualities which will improve your ability as a doctor.

REFEREES

Always ask your referees if they are willing to act as such, and let them know what job you will be using their name for. Open references are not usual in the UK. If you have not seen your referee for some time, send a copy of your updated CV for their file. This is the only time a photo may be useful, as it can be a memory jogger, distinguishing you from the other students that they have supervised. When you get the job do let them know, and say thank you for acting as a referee. This is a courtesy and will put you in a good light – they will know where you have gone, and you can always approach them again for the next job application.

Remember to keep updating your CV and keep copies of all the papers and reports you publish, as you are likely to be questioned on them during future interviews. Once you have generated your full-length CV, generate a much shorter one (two pages), as this is often the limit for anything non-medical for which you may apply. Make sure you submit a covering letter with your CV, which should state your reasons for applying for the specific job in question. You should also state any dates when you definitely can't attend an interview.

CV EXAMPLES

How not to do it

CURRICULUM VITAE
Name: Eliza Doolittle (Miss)
Address: Flat 2, Denmark House, Denmark Hill, London
Home: The Grange, Somewhere, County, SW3 2BR
DoB: 29/5/76
Status: single

EDUCATION
The Best School for Girls, Somewhere, County

GCSE English Language	A
English literature	A
Art	A*
Geography	B
Maths	A*
German	B
French	B
Double science	A*
GCE A chemistry	A
Physics	A
Biology	B
1994–	King's College Medical School MBBS
1998	BSc (hons) 2.1

WORK EXPERIENCE
1995 – The Stables, Somewhere, County. Helped with the stables.
1996 – Berlin. Playgroup worker.
1998 – KCL Immunology Dept. Laboratory work.

INTERESTS
I still enjoy painting. I like walking, riding and travelling. I can use computers.

REFEREES

Miss Sharp	Mr Hound
The Best School for Girls	The Stables
Somewhere	Somewhere
County	County
SW1 2BR	
Something better	

Comments: A high waste of space! GCSEs don't need to be listed, just summarized. A levels can be all on one line. There is very little about the MBBS or BSc – more relevant to an application for an elective or foundation post. Referees are not recent or relevant. The whole effect is childish.

Eliza Doolittle

Flat 2	Tel: 020-7123-4986
Sweden House	email: <u>eliza.doolittle@scl.ac.uk</u>
St Pancras Hill	Date of birth: 29 May 1976

Education:

1994–   **Superior College Medical School, London**
Intercalated BSc in Basic Medical Sciences and Anatomy   (2.1)
(Supported by the Muller Award for best second-year female anatomy student)
Research project: Immunological fixation of *H. pylorii* in gastric aspirate from children.
Thomas Cutting Prize for best female first-year clinical student.

1987–1994   **The Best School for Girls, Somewhere**
A levels in Chemistry (A), Physics (A) and Biology (B)
9 GCSEs 4A*, 2A and 3B
Sixth-form Science Prize

Undergraduate experience:

Exam results – specifically for electives; not necessary for foundation applications.

Hospital attachments – specifically for electives; not necessary for foundation applications.

Electives/SSMs:

1999	Elective
	Department of General Medicine, University Hospital of Berlin, Germany.
	Attended ward rounds, outpatient clinics and student teaching sessions. Also attended Accident and Emergency Department and Paediatric clinics.
1998	**Student Selected Modules included**
	Department of Cardiology, Great Ormond Street Hospital for Sick Children.
	Attended ward rounds and outpatient clinics. A library-based project was done as follow-up, looking specifically at cardiovascular disease in children.

Research/audit projects:

During my MBBS I carried out an audit on epilepsy for a local GP practice and several literature reviews for essays.

During my BSc I carried out a laboratory research project in the Immunology Department of Superior College. The findings were analysed using a variety of computer packages and the work was supported by a literature review. This was continued as a summer placement and the findings are now in press.

Career objectives:

My long-term plans are to pursue a career in paediatric medicine. This has affected my choice of summer jobs. In 1995 I worked at a riding stables, where I was responsible for two afternoon sessions per week with physically and mentally handicapped riders. This taught me patience, empathy, and the importance of challenge in improving the quality of life. In 1996 I worked in Berlin at a holiday camp for disabled children, where I was responsible for arranging and supervising their play. I learned the need for understanding while working in a foreign language.

Comment: Could be much shorter

Medically related work experience:
1997   **SCL Immunology Department:** This was a continuation of my degree project with a view to publishing my findings.

Other experience:
1998   **Travelling in Inner Mongolia:** I was part of a team of UK riders carrying a sponsored ride to visit local schools to teach English to the students.

Skills and interests:
German – fluent

Side-saddle riding (National Junior Champion – 1994). Still ride for enjoyment

Drums – play in College Orchestra and Med Soc Rock Band

Referees:
One from medical school and one from BSc project supervisor or hospital attachment (usually only two are required).

For F1 and F2/SHO posts

Warning:
This CV is not perfect and should only be used as a guideline for the production of your own (used with permission of The Careers Group, University of London).

Personal details
Name

Address   Telephone no. and email address

Nationality (if foreign-sounding name)   Marital status

GMC registration number   MDU number

Education and qualifications
Medical school

School

A

GCS

Awards

Employment and experience
Present position
Detailed responsibility, leadership, new experience
Interpersonal skills
Teaching experience
Previous in reverse chronological order
(In PRHO detail: firms and cross-disciplinary skills)

Procedures

Courses

Research/audit

Presentations – grand rounds

Publications – Vancouver style: author, the full title, the title of
the journal or book, the place of publication and the publisher
(books only), the year, volume, page numbers

Electives

Career plans (include how this post fits with your plans)

Interests/activities

Other skills

Referees (remember to contact them in writing first, and
include a job description and recent CV to help them)

SHO and SpR posts

A CV for SHO and SpR posts as suggested by the Royal College
of Surgeons (England) (CV proforma reproduced courtesy of
Royal College of Surgeons of England©)

Name
Address – Provide a permanent and a contact address and
telephone number

Date of birth   Gender

(Age – saves the shortlisted doing the sums)

Nationality   Marital status

Education
Name of medical school and dates
Name of schools and dates

Registration GMC number, MDU number and NTN (if SpR)

Degrees and diplomas

Prizes and distinctions: Don't worry if you haven't got any

Present post

Career plans

Previous appointments
Dates, number of months/years, grade hospital consultant
worked for

Eventually a summary may be a useful extension, e.g.

General surgery		PRHO 6 months
SHO		6 months
Vascular	SHO	6 months
SpR		24 months

Experience: Details of special experience under subheadings,
i.e. breast, endocrine, vascular, colorectal, upper GI, etc.
Also, a summary of operative experience, i.e. assistant,
personally assisted, unsupervised – as in logbook.

Teaching
Undergraduate
Postgraduate
Nurse
Also any teaching presentation courses attended

Management: Management experience
Can be very simple, such as arranging lists, arranging
admissions. Include things such as Mess President, etc.
Management courses attended

Audit: You should have personal experience of audit and its
principles, as it often crops up at interview. Think of
converting your audit into a publication.

Research: Give details of the research done: this section may be the one that distinguishes you from all the other candidates.

Publications: 'Submitted to...' is OK. 'In preparation' is looked on with greater scepticism.

Publications should be quoted properly, as some interviewers will read the paper.

Use Vancouver style: author, the full title, the title of the journal or book, the place of publication and the publisher (books only) the year, volume, page numbers.

Papers read at learned societies: You need a rate of converting presentations into papers, otherwise the question of perseverance and staying power may be raised.

Membership of societies: Usually professional and those you are elected to, rather than the BMA, for example, which you join by paying a subscription. Membership of some societies will be expected for some specialties, i.e. gastroenterology.

Other interests: Only needs to be brief, but it does need to show that you have a life outside surgery. If your main passion is long-distance sailing, or one that will keep you away for weeks, it does not necessarily have to be confessed here!

Referees: Give the number requested in the advert. Supplying more or fewer suggests a mailshot application not tailored to the job applied for.

APPLICATION FORMS

More and more posts require that you complete an application form; this includes applications for Foundation Schools. Most forms have instructions on how the form should be filled in – these should be followed precisely. If it says black ink, using blue ink gives the selectors a reason for rejecting your application. Do not append a CV unless it says you can – an unwanted CV is binned! If you have added a CV, try not to write 'see CV' in every box – it irritates the reader and makes you look lazy, as they have to search the CV every time for the information they require. Remember, all application forms are legal documents that are signed to say they are true. If you lie on the form and are found out by your employer, they are within their rights to terminate your employment immediately and can report the incident to the GMC, which would seriously affect your future job applications.

A job description and a person specification usually accompany an application from. The job description is self-explanatory – it describes the job you are applying for – but a few words on the person specification may be helpful.

A person specification is usually presented in table format with three columns: the criteria, 'essential' and then 'desirable'. Essential criteria are absolutely necessary to fulfil the job requirements. The desirable criteria are a wish list that the perfect applicant would also have. An MBBS or equivalent is essential to all medical jobs, and so would be placed in the 'essential' column. A BSc may be desirable but it is not essential to practise as a doctor; it would therefore be in the 'desirable' column. Other criteria are also divided this way.

Alongside the criteria are a series of codes, e.g. AF, Refs. These are how the criteria will be assessed – in this instance by the application form and from the referees. This is useful information, because if the only place something is assessed is the application form, then you must ensure that it has been covered on the form.

As well as personal and biographical information, forms may have a blank page for additional information. Here you cover information that is essential to the application apart from the person specification. Usually this section has some instruction at the top of the page, and often you are asked to include why you want this post. However, more and more forms are now assessing competencies, so don't be surprised to be asked about teamwork, stress management, your understanding of clinical governance, audit, organizational and other skills. Examples of these forms can be found on the regional Deanery websites under the relevant level of job information, as can the person specifications. It is also useful to look at the requirements of the next level up, to understand what you need to achieve to be successful at your next stage of applications. These sections can take considerable time to complete, so don't leave your application to the last minute. Do expect to take at least 8 hours to write your CV or fill out an application form. This is time well spent, as it affects the rest of your life.

FURTHER READING

Chambler AF *et al.* A model curriculum vitae: what are the trainers looking for? *Hospital Medicine* 1998; **59**: 324–6.
O'Brien E. Prepare a curriculum vitae. In: Reece D, ed. *How To Do It*. Vol 1. London: BMJ Publishing Group, 1995.
Royal College of Surgeons information for SHOs. http://www.rcseng.ac.uk

13

HOW TO BE SUCCESSFUL AT INTERVIEWS

Sonia Hutton-Taylor

INTRODUCTION

Few people truly relish being interviewed. However, as a professional person you are likely to go through a number of interviews in your life. These may be for:

- Job applications for the various grades and posts in your clinical career.
- Promotions or additional roles once you are well established in your primary career.
- To build a parallel career in non-clinical areas, such as publishing or business.
- For the purposes of career change.
- Scholarships, prizes, travel awards and grants.
- Unpaid posts on committees or charities you feel strongly about.
- Sabbatical applications.
- Informal interviews (where you might not be aware you are being interviewed).
- Medicolegal cases.

Interview skills also overlap with presentation skills and viva examination skills, in that all three are 'performing in front of others under pressure', and each is probably borne with some degree of nerves.

Some important promotions, awards or entries into new directions are not decided by interview, of course. There are other methods. For example, more than one medical school used to select students without interview but on grades and UCAS reports. One medical school now selecting for a specific mature graduate programme is using a wide range of processes in addition to interview, including an essay, a science examination and psychometric testing.

It has been said by certain experienced medical interview panellists that interviews as a process are flawed, and are not sufficient to decide whether a person is suitable for a job. This is probably why for many years in the commercial world graduate and senior management posts required candidates to attend a 2-day formal 'assessment centre', where a range of tests and methodologies are used to help weed out the unsuitable and identify the best candidates.

Traditional medical interviews are starting to be supplemented with additional selection methods (see below). But whatever your views on the 'standard' interview, these thrilling or excruciating experiences (depending on your attitude and skill) can still decide important aspects of your future, your income, your success, your job satisfaction and possibly even your health – all good reasons why you need to learn how to handle them.

It is difficult but necessary to strike a balance between coming across better than you actually are and stating your case as best you can. Getting the right balance between these two extremes – i.e. honesty/realism and selling/ promotion – is the key skill in doing well at interviews, but it is one that is rarely tackled comprehensively.

There are three typical approaches to interview:

- Head in the sand – hoping it will go away, or that no-one will turn up on the day, or that somehow you can 'wing' it.
- Laissez faire – doing a bit of preparation and thinking about some questions beforehand – usually the night before.
- Focused – using a structured, critical, developmental and considered strategy that begins weeks (if not months) before the interview.

The third option is what this chapter is all about. For the sake of simplicity we will be referring mainly to job interviews, but the principles are the same for each and every type of interview.

THE PLACE TO START

There is a good, reliable approach to interviews, which can be divided into three sections – before, during and after.

Before

A recent straw poll of doctors seeking jobs revealed a big variation in how much preparation individuals do for interviews, ranging from 'reading a CV on the way to the interview' to 'a 6-week preparation'.

Each person is different in the amount of time they should devote to interview preparation and planning. The time to invest is directly proportional to the difficulty experienced in past interview situations, or to how nervous or lacking in confidence you think you will be.

In severe 'interview phobia' cases – for those with really poor self-promotion skills, or where a really prized job is on the horizon – interview training with an expert could start several months beforehand, so that there is plenty of time for practice and improvement before the big day.

Think about what tasks a future job may hold. If you don't feel instantly that you have oodles of experience in the skills you will need, then not only must you then formulate a sensible answer to counter any searching questions that may come up on this but if you start to do all this far enough in advance you can also start to address any apparent areas of insufficiency. For example, if you apply to do research with an eminent professor for your elective, you should learn exactly what his/her research involves and what directions it has taken. In any interview, they would want to know why you have chosen them to work with.

What preparation?

The aim of your preparation should be 'to learn how to sell yourself in a positive light in relation to the post without overblowing your own trumpet and sounding arrogant or big headed'. Easier said than done. . . .

The best way to achieve this elusive balance is:

1. To know yourself and your skills, experience and career aims.
2. To be able to articulate fluently and comfortably.
3. To know the job and the career/specialty.
4. To be able to converse sensibly about the responsibilities of the post, how you might fit into the unit or team, and what you will bring to the post – i.e. selling.
5. To anticipate as many questions or topic areas as possible in advance.
6. To write down your answers to these; read, rehearse, and plan around them.

Doing insufficient homework and analysis on any one of these six areas could make you miss a post that you were in fact ideally suited to. Thus dealing with all of these except, for example, number three, would mean you could fall down significantly on what the promotion will actually mean in terms of new roles for you, and you will look quite naïve if you can't converse in the current hot topics in your specialty. Let's deal with these areas in more detail.

Know yourself

This is potentially a lifetime's work, of course. Interview panels are often aware that to be an effective and productive member of a team a person must know himself or herself well – personality, good and bad points, values, motivations, skills, limitations and more. Interviews can quite easily reveal a person who is not in touch with these areas, and if someone else is, other things being equal, they will get the job. People who do not know themselves well have a tendency to either answer questions in a more arrogant fashion or to grossly undersell themselves. Thus self-understanding and insight are often crucial to good performance in interviews.

Virtually all questions have an element of self-revelation in how you answer them, but there are some more specific questions designed to winkle out information about you as a person. These would include questions such as:

● What is your greatest strength/weakness?
● How would you describe yourself?
● What interaction with patients do you find most challenging?

Articulate fluently

Not everyone can think fast off the top of their head. So, getting practice in actually speaking your answers out loud and getting used to talking about yourself in positive terms can be invaluable. Feedback from others (colleagues, family, friends and tutors) in dummy interviews can help you to start honing some good phrases and comments that you feel comfortable with.

One reason people don't come across well at interview is 'nerves'. Some apprehension is normal, but for many people their ability to be coherent and relaxed is severely compromised by anxiety and its manifestations (sweating, fidgeting, expression, nervous laughter, stumbling over responses, blurting out daft comments, and more). Overcoming anxiety at interviews for some people is relatively easy, but for others might require months of work.

A key skill is to listen very carefully to the question and not to rush into an answer. Many candidates do not answer the question they have just been asked. If a question is not clear in its remit, then ask a question back to clarify it.

The key methods are:

- Good preparation.
- Gaining experience in all types of public speaking situations at every opportunity.
- Practice (e.g. with dictaphone, mirror, buddy, boss or video).
- Specific techniques, such as deep breathing, and so on.

Know the job

All too often people see a job advertised which asks for a CV to be sent in. The CV is then sent off without the individual doing any background research into the job, the employing organization or the department. A more comprehensive approach to tailoring a CV after learning more about the post may increase the chances of being shortlisted, but if you get to an interview, this becomes an essential part of your preparation.

There are many ways to find out more about a post:

- Speak to the departmental secretary.
- Speak to the current post holder.
- Speak to the regional adviser in the specialty, where possible.
- Go to the organization's website.
- Speak to the HR department and ask for a copy of the annual report.
- Obtain and read carefully the job description, person specification, and all other information that may be sent to you.

Do this comprehensive research and you will start to see which parts of your past are particularly relevant to the post, and how you can specifically contribute to the department. You can also tactfully interject your extensive knowledge of the post and organization into any pre-interview visits, and occasionally make reference to key issues for the department or organization in your answers to questions.

Selling

Doctors are notoriously bad at or uncomfortable with the whole issue of 'selling'. This is probably because in the public sector an overt 'sale' rarely, if ever, takes place, and the only exposure doctors get to selling is via drug reps, which can taint their perception of selling. Doctors themselves can be perfectionists, some of whom generally feel they are never doing as well as they could be, and consequently tend to do themselves down rather than up (when even a middle ground would suffice!).

Selling yourself at interview generally involves first having prepared in advance what you think are your key selling points, becoming well-versed in talking about them with ease, and then seeing opportunities within the questions asked to expand upon your skills and introduce them into the answer. This is not something most people can do without some considerable thought well in advance.

Anticipate

It can be a great idea to keep an expanding list of interview questions gleaned from your own common sense, from reading the medical press, asking those who have just been to an interview, your own interviews and asking those on interview panels which questions tend to be answered badly. See Appendix II for a selection to get you started – but you can't beat keeping a list of your own.

Write it down

Once you have this list you can start writing possible answers. There is no space in this chapter to cover all the questions that could be asked in every specialty or every interview situation. For this reason, we will deal with the principles involved. There is also another reason we are not listing hundreds of questions and answers, and that is that over time the questions asked tend to change – if for no other reason than that the panels start to realize that past questions used are now generally answered rather too glibly by the candidates (which suggests that interview training courses have now absorbed these, and that the questions are too commonplace to be helpful in distinguishing between well-prepared candidates). Furthermore, new questions are being generated all the time as medical and healthcare politics or agendas change – it is therefore more important to learn the principles of how to deal with questions, rather than memorize specific 'perfect' answers.

A good approach to answering potential questions during preparation is to write the answer down, rather than trying to keep things in your head. Once your answer is there in black and white you can then analyse it, try to refine it or, if you are concerned about what to say, seek feedback from others.

Sample approach to a question

Q: What is your greatest strength?
The approach to any question is to think 'What is it they could be after here?' and then 'What aspect of myself can I sell in a positive light?', followed by 'How can I phrase the most important points I want to get across succinctly and effectively?'

In this question, the panel are trying to see whether you know yourself well, whether you can produce a response that reaches a sensible mature person's balance between humility and genuine self appreciation, and whether you can relate this strength to the workplace and back it up in terms of hard evidence. If you had not thought this through well in advance your answer might be a tad brief:
A: I am an excellent team player.

Not only is this answer short, it does not lead the panel into any useful conclusion about you: it is bland, unsupported, and bordering on bragging. In summary, it is not good 'selling'.

At the other extreme might be a whole load of unfocused, repetitive, rambling waffly chitchat:

A: I have always found it very hard to pin down one strength, as most people, it seems to me, have more than one area they could mention if pressed. If I had a gun held to my head I would probably have to say that I do get along well with others and like to have good relationships with my colleagues from all disciplines. I really like working with people and find working in a caring environment really rewarding. I don't know if that is my greatest strength, but it is the one that comes to mind most readily as it is really important to me, and I always seem to fit in quite easily and get on well with everyone I work with. Having a friendly atmosphere at work is important and I do my best to ensure that I contribute to that. I like working with nurses, porters, lab staff, doctors, ward clerks – everyone really, etc., etc. (When are they going to stop?!).

A more focused yet positive 'sales' answer with more balance might be:

A: I think my greatest strength is probably an ability to get on well with a wide range of personalities and professionals. In this specialty, multidisciplinary working is increasingly important, and respecting the experience of other team members is crucial to effectiveness and morale. I have twice been elected as a representative for junior doctors, and I suspect this is because I tend to naturally take on board others' opinions and try to make each person feel valued. But a greatest strength of course can also be a greatest weakness.

This answer shows that that the person has thought about this issue and knows themselves well enough to realize how they interact in a work situation and what influences their effectiveness. It shows some good people management skills. It also gives some evidence to back up the points made.

At the end it makes an attempt at 'setting up the next question'. This is a technique that can help to influence where an interview goes. Some panels have a strict list of questions they can ask, but the way in which this answer ends might just be too tempting. The next question is naturally, 'So how is your greatest strength also your greatest weakness?' – which, of course, if you have also prepared well is just what you want.

The other key point is that any answer has to be owned by the person. For example, it's no good adopting the above answer if this is not *your* greatest strength. In addition, even if your greatest strength is getting along with others, the context in which you do so will be unique to you, and so your answer should also be unique. This method of tailoring answers to your own personality and abilities is crucial, and it is why we have not made this chapter a long list of questions with 'perfect' answers (however, a reference list of questions asked at SHO and SpR level interviews is provided in Appendix II).

- Be clear about why this is your job.
- What is special about you?
- What does the interview panel want to hear (what are their person specification criteria)? Put yourself in their shoes – would they want you as a colleague? What is important to them?
- How do you think you want to behave and feel during the interview?
- Know what your weaknesses are and how you plan to overcome them.
- Don't forget to read health media and journals in and around your specialty in the months leading up to the interview.

Rehearse

Once you have produced answers to your list of questions, rehearse them over and over again. Try to get a senior doctor with whom you are not too familiar to give you a mock interview (this will simulate the pressure of the interview). Make a video of yourself if possible, and observe and critique your own posture, body language and clarity during a mock interview.

ON THE DAY AND DURING AN INTERVIEW

The blindingly obvious (but not to all, it seems!):

- Be sure to get a good night's sleep – if an on-call rota is unfavourable, try to swap with a colleague.
- Have a final look through your CV and make sure you know it inside out.
- Clean nails, hair and clothes (take a spare tie).
- Take any documents with you that might be relevant – but don't keep them on your lap: have a case or folder that you put down beside you when you sit down, so you don't fiddle with it.
- Take your mobile and know who to contact if you are running late (turn it off before you go in for the actual interview).
- Arrive with plenty of time – far better to be an hour early than five minutes late! Lateness does nothing for nerves, and if you're early there is time to practise those relaxation techniques!
- Sit elegantly. Many people have poor or casual posture that increases the chances of revealing nerves. For example, a leg crossed can encourage a 'wobbly' or bouncing foot, which can be very distracting. Clasped hands have the tendency to fidget. So keep both feet on the floor, hands one on each thigh and back in contact with the chair. It is fine to raise one or both hands in certain explanations to complement your answer, but then put them back down in the 'rest' position (i.e. don't keep waving them about).
- Smile – but don't do a Jim Carrey! Overuse of smiling generally denotes an unassertive, apologetic personality,

or else nerves. A funereal face may hint at a person who takes themselves a bit too seriously, or that they are nervous too. A generally straight face with the occasional smile in appropriate places is a good balance.

● Make plenty of eye contact. This is of course a big challenge where mega-panels (6+) are involved, but it is OK to make the main eye contact with the person asking the question, giving occasional glances to the other members of the panel.

● Answer the question asked and don't trail off into completely different issues.

● When answering a question, try to keep your options open, allow yourself room for manoeuvre, and give balanced answers to difficult problems (recognize both sides of an argument).

● This interview is not the time to express controversial views.

● Don't argue with the panel under any circumstances, but do speak with enthusiasm.

● For some questions that require a longer explanation, you often need to give a structure to your answer at the start, so you lay a foundation and then follow it through with the details; this shows you can think and explain things clearly. Always try to present your answers concisely and be aware of speed and tone (don't rush because of nerves: take your time, be confident and assert yourself).

● You are more likely to score highly by delivering several concise answers over a range of subjects, rather than spending all your time answering just one question (especially the first one). This ability to know when to stop talking is important (don't ramble on: instead, go for cool professionalism with enthusiasm).

● If you feel you have answered a question fully, don't be tempted to keep talking, even if there is a brief period of silence with which you feel uncomfortable.

● If you feel your last answer was poor, put it behind you and focus on the next question: you may be able to redeem yourself.

ALTERNATIVE SELECTION METHODS

There is an increasing range of ways to differentiate between candidates, and it is worth being aware that interviews *per se* are no longer the only method. The alternatives may include:

- In-tray/out-tray exercises
- Presentations
- Written challenges
- Role play
- Observed team activities
- Formal assessment centres or 'days'
- Psychometric testing.

When you are invited to interview it is likely that you will be fully informed of any additional methods to be used in selection, but it is worth clarifying this. Like interviews, these methods are designed to find out more about the candidate, particularly on issues such as teamworking, leadership, decision-making, interpersonal skills, confidence and general common sense. Once again, the night before the interview is not the time to attempt to fashion such skills, as they need to be addressed in training and personal development plans well in advance of interviews.

AFTER AN INTERVIEW

Many people breathe a sigh of relief as they walk out the door of the interview room and instantly forget all that went on. This is a mistake, mainly because if there is any chance that you may not have got the job you need to do some audit and review of what has just happened. If you don't do this, painful though it may be, you will be missing an invaluable learning opportunity to improve your approach at the next interview.

So what should you do?

First, it is important to jot down as many questions as you can recall, and also the answers that you gave. If you leave it a few hours many of these will be lost forever. Writing them down immediately after you leave the interview room will improve your chances of remembering a fair number.

Having written down the questions and answers, try to write an honest appraisal of yourself in this interview and ask yourself the following:

- Were there any questions that went particularly well?
- Were there any that went badly?
- Some of these questions and answers you will have prepared well for, but how did you do under fire?
- Did you feel that each answer was received well, or did they seem to be looking for something additional?
- Did the interview have a relaxed happy feel to it, or did you sense tension or hostility?
- Did you do or say anything that you would try to repeat or avoid in future interviews?
- How did the interview begin and end? Was each satisfactory?

Get that feedback!

For many posts decisions are given on the same day, and sometimes very soon after the interview. So the next stage is to attempt to get some feedback from the interview panel. This is absolutely vital if you did not get the job. However, interview panels are often tired after the interviewing, not always aware of how to give constructive and helpful feedback and may not have the time or inclination to do so. Obtaining feedback can therefore be extraordinarily difficult, but here are some tips for getting at least something.

Try to phrase your request for feedback in a constructive and positive way for yourself. If you enjoyed your interview, say so (but don't lie, as it will probably be clear to the panel that you were squirming and sweating if you were). State that you were naturally disappointed but keen to know where you could do better, and why you were not the top choice.

Try to evade and parry comments such as 'You were overqualified', or 'You did really well, but there was somebody just a bit more suitable' by replying 'Well I realized that, but I wondered if you could point out any areas where I could do better at interview, or any areas in my career where I should pay more attention?' If they repeat their vague unhelpful comments, merely repeat your question a little more enthusiastically so they realize they can't escape. Try to do this as soon after the interview as is humanly possible. If interviewers have just seen 20 people their recall of your performance may not last long.

Even with the best assertiveness in the world, some interviewers are simply not aware of how important feedback can be to the unsuccessful candidate's career. Even if they suggest they think you are unlikely to succeed in this career route with your given skills and experience, this feedback – albeit painful – can be invaluable, in that it can either stiffen resolve and focus the mind, or it can help one come to terms with the need to seek some objective career guidance, and perhaps to look at a wider range of options.

GETTING BETTER AT INTERVIEWS

If you have followed the advice above and still have no job (or scholarship or committee position, etc.), there are a number of ways to approach this, depending on the cause of your lack of success. These include:

- Public speaking training and practice.
- Selling skills training (so that you can adopt a more balanced approach to selling yourself if you are not comfortable with doing this).
- Seeking interview training.
- Get friends and colleagues to interview or video you, and ask them to be brutal!

Interviews and your performance in them can make or break your career path. It is perhaps not entirely fair that those who can master them with ease do better on the job front. However, although interviews are not foolproof ways of getting the best person for a post, they are still the core method and are used with or without additional methods of selection. So, developing a strategy to do well in them is a sensible thing to do. To avoid the issue of interviews altogether in the hope it will go away, or that somehow you will 'wing' it, is failure to address a key element of career progression. Try to learn from failure, and remember that factors beyond your control may have clinched the decision. Finally, remember that nobody has ever failed at anything unless that is the last time they are going to try.

FURTHER READING

1:1 and telephone interview/self promotion/job-hunt training. Medical Forum. http://www.medicalforum.com

Discussion groups on jobs and interviews. http://www. doctors.net

e-course in interview skills. Medical Forum. http://www. medicalforum.com

Mumford C. *The Medical Interview: Secrets for Success.* Oxford: Blackwell Science, 2001.

Past articles on interview topics – BMJ Careers. http://www. bmjcareers.com

Various workshops/courses (advertised in BMJ Careers). http://www.bmjcareers.com

APPENDIX 1

SOURCES OF FUNDING FOR YOUR INTERCALATED BSc AND YOUR ELECTIVE

Go to www.yourmedicalcareer.com to get the most up-to-date list of awards available and download their applications forms directly from the site.

FUNDING YOUR INTERCALATED BSC

Always read the full eligibility criteria for each award.
(*See* Table A1)

FUNDING YOUR ELECTIVE

The following awards are available for elective students (please note that amounts are approximate and subject to change, and please make sure you read their individual eligibility criteria)
(*See* Table A2)

OTHER NON-SPECIFIC SOURCES OF POTENTIAL SUPPORT

- Your university or medical school awards – there will be many, so research these at the earliest opportunity and consult staff and older students.
- *University Scholarships and Awards* by Brian Heap. Published by Trotman.
- Enquire about hardship funds and hardship loans at your medical school registry.

Table A1 Sources of funding for intercalated BSc

Awarding Body	Amount	Annual Application Deadline
The Wellcome Trust www.wellcome.ac.uk/en/1/biosfgcdpfunsumvac.html	£165 per week for up to 8 weeks	26 March
The Health Foundation (formerly the PPP Foundation) www.health.org.uk/ourawards/otherawards/index.cfm?id=19	£6000	Nominated by your Dean (ask at your registry)
The Physiological Society www.physoc.org/grants/full_details/index.asp?ID=5	Up to £1200	30 April
Vandervell Foundation (020 7248 9045) Vandervell Foundation, Bridge House, 181 Queen Victoria Street, London EC4V 4DD	Around £300	None
Mary Datchelor Trust (020 7623 7041) The Clothworkers' Foundation, Clothworkers' Hall, Dunster Court, Mincing Lane, London EC3R 7AH	£500	None
Gilchrist Educational Trust Mary Trevelyan Hall, 10 York Terrace East, London NW1 4PT	Variable	Variable
National Pressure Ulcer Advisory Panel www.npuap.org/research_award.html	Variable	1 November
European Wound Management Association www.ewma.org/english/english.htm	Variable (around £500)	May
European Society of Vascular Surgery www.esvs.org/grants/research.asp	Variable	31 May
British Association of Dermatologists www.bad.org.uk/doctors/fellowships/	£500	20 March
Pathological Society of Great Britain and Ireland www.pathsoc.org.uk	Variable	1 March
Association of Anaesthetists of Great Britain and Ireland	Up to £300	7 January

Table A2 Sources of funding for elective

Awarding Body	Amount	Annual Application Deadline
British Geriatrics Society www.bgs.org.uk/grants/annette/granttest.htm#ms	Up to £500	None
The Royal College of Surgeons of England – Preiskel Elective Prize in Surgery www.rcseng.ac.uk/surgical/research/awards/preiskel_html	£500	March
Vandervell Foundation (020 7248 9045) Vandervell Foundation, Bridge House, 181 Queen Victoria Street, London EC4V 4DD	Around £300	None
Mary Datchelor Trust (020 7623 7041) The Clothworkers' Foundation, Clothworkers' Hall, Dunster Court, Mincing Lane, London EC3R 7AH	£500	None
British Association of Plastic Surgeons www.baps.co.uk/education/assoc-awards.htm	£500	31 December
British Microcirculation Society www.microcirculation.org.uk/LVG.html	Up to £800	31 January or 30 June
Cancer Research UK http://science.cancerresearchuk.org/gapp/?version = 3	£1000	February (Nominated by the Dean)
Pathological Society of Great Britain and Ireland www.pathsoc.org.uk	Up to £75 per week	31 May
British Association of Dermatologists www.bad.org.uk/doctors/fellowships/	£500	20 March
British Nutrition Foundation (BNF/Nestle Bursary Scheme and the Denis Burkitt Study Award) www.nutrition.org.uk/	£500 or £750	31 January

(continued)

Table A2 (continued)

Awarding Body	Amount	Annual Application Deadline
British Association of Forensic Medicine www.shef.ac.uk/~bafm/stu.html	£200	Not stated
Association of Anaesthetists of Great Britain and Ireland www.aagbi.org.uk/	£750	7 January
Section of Anaesthesia at the Royal Society of Medicine www.rsm.ac.uk	£500	2 February
Section of Accident and Emergency at the Royal Society of Medicine www.rsm.ac.uk	£500	31 March
The Physiological Society www.physoc.org/grants/full_details/index.asp?ID = 5	Up to £1200	30 April
Royal College of Physicians (The Oscar Reginald Lewis Wilson Studentship) www.rcplondon.ac.uk/college/conf_fellowships.htm	£250	Nominated by the Dean by end of March
Diabetes UK www.diabetes.org.uk/research/grants/types.htm#travel	Up to £250	1 month before you are due to go
European Society of Vascular Surgery www.esvs.org/grants/research.asp	Variable	31 May
The Wellcome Trust www.wellcome.ac.uk/en/1/biosfgcdpfunsumsep.html	£1000	1 May
British Medical and Dental Students Trust Request an application form from: Secretary, British Medical and Dental Students' Trust, Mackintosh House, 120 Blythswood, Glasgow, G2 4EH	£200–£600	Apply as early as possible
GlaxoSmithKline Medical Fellowship	£1000	31 May

European Wound Management Association www.ewma.org/english/english.htm	Variable (around £500)	May
National Pressure Ulcer Advisory Panel www.npuap.org/research_award.html	Variable	1 November
Gilchrist Educational Trust Mary Trevelyan Hall, 10 York Terrace East, London NW1 4PT	Variable	Variable
Lepra (The British Leprosy Relief Association) www.lepra.org.uk/projects/electives.shtml	Variable	6 months prior to your elective
Your Local Rotary Club www.rotary.org/foundation/educational/amb_scho/prospect/index.html	Variable	Variable
Child Health Research Appeal Trust Registrar, The Institute of Child Health, University of London, 30 Guilford Street, London WC1N 1EH	125/week	Variable
British Society for Haematology Student Scholarships Scientific Secretary, British Society for Haematology, 2 Carlton House Terrace, London SW1Y 5AF	£600	No closing date
The National Birthday Trust Fund Mary Stanton, The National Birthday Trust Fund, 27 Sussex Place, Regent's Park, London NW1 4SP.	£250	Variable
Clegg Scholarship StudentBMJ, BMA House, Tavistock Square, London WC1H 9TR	£600	3 November
Medical Women's Federation Student Elective Bursaries Dr J Wells, 62 Denbigh Street, London SW1V 2EX	£300	31 May

(continued)

Table A2 (continued)

Awarding Body	Amount	Annual Application Deadline
Milupa Student Elective Grant Fund Mr T L Bell, Managing Director, Milupa Ltd, Milupa House, Uxbridge Road, Hillingdon, Middlesex UV10 0NE	£500	31 May
St Francis Leprosy Guild Secretary, St Francis Leprosy Guild, 21 The Boultons, London SW10 9SU	£600	Variable
Thackrah Award The Executive Secretary, Society of Occupational Medicine, 6 St Andrews Place, Regents Park, London. NW1 4LB	£1000	Variable
A H Bygott Scholarship Academic Trust Funds Committee, Senate House, Room 234, Malet Street, London WC1E 7HU.	£750	Variable
Renal Association Bursaries Secretary, Renal Association, Triangle 3 Ltd, Triangle House, Broomfield Road, London SW18 4IH	£250	Variable

- *The Grants Register.* Published by MacMillan Reference Ltd.
- The Association of Medical Research Charities www.amrc.org.uk.
- *The Charities Digest.*
- Charities Direct www.charitiesdirect.com
- NHS Info site www.rdinfo.org.uk.

FURTHER READING

Heap B. University Scholarships and Awards. Richmond: Trotman, 2002.

APPENDIX 11
QUESTIONS ASKED AT JOB INTERVIEWS

The questions below represent a sample of the potential questions that can be asked. Thinking under pressure is tough, so give yourself the best chance of success by preparing your 'spontaneous' answers in advance. Try going through these lists and have a think about each question. Then get someone to interview you asking a question from each section in random order; try to recall and recite your prepared answer in a spontaneous way, i.e. as if an interview situation.

GENERAL

- Why do you want this job?
- Why this specialty?
- Why this city/hospital?
- Why do you want to come to this region?
- Give your experience to date in jobs or posts.
- Take me through your clinical posts and career progression since qualification.
- Are there any gaps in your training to date?
- Talk us through your CV.
- What did you think of the course you attended on .... ?
- Tell me about your stamp collecting/modern dance/Olympic gold medal in judo/culinary expertise that you have mentioned in your CV.
- What skills can you bring to the job?
- Are there any gaps in your training to date?

- What do you think of your training so far?
- Why should we give you this job?
- Why should you be given the job over another candidate?
- What is your plan for the next year?
- What is your plan for the next five years?
- Where do you see yourself in five years' time?
- What are your career objectives?
- What are your ultimate career intentions?
- 'Is there anything you want to ask the panel?' (Hint: use an intelligent phrase such as, 'No, I don't think so – I have found out all I need to know already about this post and unit by visiting and talking to the junior doctors, consultants and other staff on the ward.')

CLINICAL

- What have you gained as a senior house officer (SHO)?
- What did you gain from jobs before entering this specialty?
- Give an example of where you've prioritized clinical need.
- Would you rather work in a shift pattern or a traditional 24-hour on-call pattern?
- Give an example of where you've had to work as a member of a multidisciplinary team.
- Give two clinical situations that have helped you improve your practice.
- Tell us of an interesting case you have handled recently.
- What is the most challenging clinical situation you have met?
- Tell me about a memorable case where you learned something new.
- You've done a locum appointment in training post – what was the most important step up you had to deal with compared with being a senior house officer?
- What could you do to improve the organization and running of your current workplace environment?
- Would you be happy being an average consultant?
- What characteristics make a good consultant?

- Tell me about the most recent paper you've read which will change your day-to-day clinical practice?
- What invasive procedures have you performed and what complications have you encountered?
- What measures do you use to obtain informed consent for the procedures you do?
- When was the last time you rang your consultant?
- Tell me about a situation where your communication skills did not succeed in getting something done.

You may be asked a specific clinical management question relevant to the post, for example management of acute asthma, seizures, arrhythmia, etc.

SPECIALTY

- Why do you want to train in this specialty?
- What are your aims for your time on the training scheme?
- If you could improve the specialty training scheme in one way, what would you choose to do?
- What are the main trends in the specialty at the moment?
- What complications of procedure X should you be aware of?
- Tell me about the evidence base for the treatment of condition X.
- Who was (important person in history of specialty)?

ACADEMIC

- Take me through your academic achievements since arriving at medical school.
- If you were planning your own medical curriculum, what would you alter?
- Do you have any prizes, and did you find going for them useful?
- Research – why haven't you done any? If you have done any, summarize your research as briefly as possible.

- How did you organize your research project?
- Did your supervisor write your grant application?
- How much of your research is your own design and how much is guided by your supervisor?
- What did you learn from your research?
- What have you gained from your publications?
- What is your best paper and why?
- Tell me about an interesting paper you've read in the past three months.
- Do you want to do further research?
- How have you kept your clinical skills and knowledge up to date during your research?
- Do you think research helps a doctor be a good doctor?
- Should every trainee in this specialty undertake research?
- Should research be carried out at tertiary centres, or do district general hospitals have a role?
- What do you understand by the term 'research governance'?

AUDIT

- What is audit?
- What audit projects have you done, and what were the results?
- What did you learn?
- Was the audit loop closed?
- What is your best and your worst audit, and why?
- What problems are there in the way SHO audit projects are carried out?

TEACHING

- What is your experience of teaching?
- What specific skills have you learned that make you a good teacher?
- Which one technique has had the biggest impact on your teaching methods?
- How do you organize a teaching session?

PERSONALITY FOCUSED

- What are your strengths?
- What are your weaknesses?
- What is the most difficult situation you have been in?
- How do you deal with difficult situations?
- How would you deal with conflict in the department?
- Do you ever lose your temper?
- What is the most stressful situation you have been in within the last six months?
- How do you cope with stress?
- How would you cope with criticism and a complaint against you?
- If you were able to do one thing that could improve the wellbeing of the world/mankind, what would you do?
- What was the most important event in your life?
- Describe yourself in as few sentences as possible.
- What are you most proud of?
- What would you do if a colleague was underperforming?
- How would you deal with a problem doctor – for example if you suspected your consultant had a drink problem?
- What is your relationship with managers like?
- What is your relationship with your colleagues like?
- If you were to start your career again, what would you change?
- Are you assertive?
- How do you organize a multidisciplinary team to work on a project?

NHS ISSUES

- What do you understand by the term clinical governance?
- Are there any problems with the implementation of clinical governance?
- What do you think of foundation hospitals?
- What do you think of NICE (National Institute of Clinical Excellence)?

- What do you think of CHAI (Commission for Healthcare Audit and Inspection)?
- What do you think of CHIMP (Centre for Health Improvement)/CHI (Commission for Health Improvement)?
- What is the Commission for Health Improvement?
- What is the role of the National Patient Safety Agency?
- What do you think of Calmanization?
- What do you understand by the term clinical risk management?
- What is a near-miss situation?
- Is the expanding role of nurses a benefit or a danger to the medical profession?
- What is appraisal?
- What do you think of the consultant contract?
- What is assessment?
- What are National Service Frameworks?
- How has the recent National Service Framework affected your hospital's practice; how is its implementation being measured?
- What are your views on NHS recruitment drives in the developing world?
- What is competence?
- What is competence-based assessment?
- What is revalidation?
- What is the NHS plan?
- What do you think of doctors' hours, the European Working Time Directive and the Hospital at Night project?
- What do you think of Modernizing Medical Careers?

MISCELLANEOUS

- What information technology skills do you possess?
- How do you organize an on-call rota?
- How would you set up a journal club?
- Talk about your elective experiences.

● What did you think of your elective?
● How do you draw the line between seeking advice versus acting independently?
● Discuss some ethical dilemmas you have been faced with.

FURTHER READING

Hutton-Taylor S. Interview questions. http://www.medicalforum. com/interview-question-bank.htm

Pickersgill T. What are the questions usually asked in interviews for senior house officer jobs? *BMJ Careers Focus* 2004; **329**: 2.

Scoote M, Elkington A, Thaventhiran J. How to prepare for your first specialist registrar interview. *BMJ Career Focus* 2004; **328**: 233–5 (web extra material).

INDEX

Note: page numbers in **bold** refer to diagrams, page numbers in *italics* refer to information contained in tables.